Application of the International Classification of Diseases to Dentistry and Stomatology

Third Edition

ICD-DA

Application of the International Classification of Diseases to Dentistry and Stomatology

Third Edition

World Health Organization
Geneva
1995

First edition 1973
Second edition 1978
Third edition 1994

WHO Library Cataloguing in Publication Data
Application of the International Classification of Diseases to dentistry and stomatology:
ICD-DA. — 3rd ed.
1.Mouth diseases — classification
2.Mouth neoplasms — classification
3.Tooth diseases — classification

ISBN 92 4 154467 8   (NLM Classification: WU 15)

The World Health Organization welcomes requests for permission to reproduce or translate its publications, in part or in full. Applications and enquiries should be addressed to the Office of Publications, World Health Organization, Geneva, Switzerland, which will be glad to provide the latest information on any changes made to the text, plans for new editions, and reprints and translations already available.

© World Health Organization 1995

The designations employed and the presentation of the material in this publication do not imply the expression of any opinion whatsoever on the part of the Secretariat of the World Health Organization concerning the legal status of any country, territory, city or area or of its authorities, or concerning the delimitation of its frontiers or boundaries.

The mention of specific companies or of certain manufacturers' products does not imply that they are endorsed or recommended by the World Health Organization in preference to others of a similar nature that are not mentioned. Errors and omissions excepted, the names of proprietary products are distinguished by initial capital letters.

Typeset in India
Printed in England
93/9818–Macmillan/Clays–8500

Contents

Preface to the third edition

On the initiative of the International Dental Federation, a meeting of consultants was convened by the World Health Organization in 1964 to consider the classification of diseases of the buccal cavity in relation to the impending Eighth (1965) Revision of the International Classification of Diseases (ICD). It was recognized that a manual and guide should be compiled to assist in the application of the ICD to dentistry and stomatology. Accordingly, a text was drafted and tested in four countries, then revised and published for general use. The first version of the *Application of the International Classification of Diseases to Dentistry and Stomatology (ICD-DA)* was issued in English in 1969, followed by publication in Spanish in 1970.[1] The first WHO edition was published in English in 1973.[2]

Publication of the Ninth Revision of ICD, which came into effect in Member States in 1978, gave rise to the second edition of ICD-DA.[3] This third edition has been prepared as a companion volume to ICD-10, the Tenth Revision of ICD.

WHO gratefully acknowledges the work done by the many national institutes and individual specialists who contributed to the preparation and revision of ICD-DA. Special acknowledgements are due to Professor I.R.H. Kramer, Emeritus Professor of Oral Pathology, University of London, London, England, and Professor J.J. Pindborg, Dental School, University of Copenhagen, Copenhagen, Denmark, who have assumed the major responsibility for the preparation of all three editions of ICD-DA.

---

[1] *Application of the International Classification of Diseases to Dentistry and Stomatology (ICD-DA)*. Copenhagen, Dental Department, University Hospital, 1969.

Clasificación internacional de enfermedades, aplicada a odontologia y estomatologia. Washington, DC, Pan American Health Organization, 1970 (PAHO Scientific Publication No. 206).

[2] *Application of the International Classification of Diseases to Dentistry and Stomatology (ICD-DA)*. Geneva, World Health Organization, 1973.

[3] *Application of the International Classification of Diseases to Dentistry and Stomatology (ICD-DA)*, 2nd ed. Geneva, World Health Organization, 1978.

Introduction

When any substantial volume of data has to be recorded, a coherent system of classifying and coding the data is essential, particularly where electronic or mechanical means of retrieval or analysis are to be used.

The *Application of the International Classification of Diseases to Dentistry and Stomatology (ICD-DA)* is intended to provide a practical and convenient basis for the classification and coding of data by all those working in the field of oral and dental disorders. It is derived directly from the Tenth Revision of the International Classification of Diseases (ICD-10),[1] and is concerned with all diseases and conditions that occur in, have manifestations in, or are associated with the oral cavity and adjacent structures.

For the purposes of ICD-DA, most of the classifications provided by ICD-10 have been subdivided and expanded; however, data from ICD-DA can be reassembled into ICD categories by simple addition. It is strongly recommended that ICD-DA be used with ICD-10 available for reference; use of ICD-10 alone is unsuitable for the following reasons:

● categories for the diseases and conditions of interest to oral health personnel are insufficiently subdivided;

● the diseases and conditions are scattered throughout the large volume, which makes its use in oral health facilities both awkward and time-consuming.

The principal objectives of ICD-DA are thus:

● to focus the attention of oral health personnel on detailed diagnosis for each patient, using a comprehensive and consistent classification of oral diseases and oral manifestations of other diseases;

---

[1] *International Statistical Classification of Diseases and Related Health Problems. Tenth revision.* Geneva, World Health Organization.
Volume 1. Tabular list. 1992
Volume 2. Instruction manual. 1993
Volume 3. Alphabetical index. 1994

- to provide a standard recording system for all oral diseases and conditions;

- by means of the recording system, to make possible the collection of data that will allow the prevalence of oral diseases and conditions to be compared at an international level.

In addition to facilitating international collaboration and exchange of information, it is hoped that the ICD-DA system will contribute substantially to the collection of epidemiological data on the rarer oral diseases, for which purpose the survey method is impracticable.

ICD-DA is of value to a wide variety of users, from governments collecting basic data to individual researchers, practitioners, and lecturers who require a convenient method for indexing their records and teaching material. It can be used in a contracted form, consisting of a relatively small number of broad headings, or in an expanded form that allows detailed analysis in areas of special interest.

The International Classification of Diseases

Readers and users of ICD-DA are referred to ICD-10 for a detailed treatment of the general principles, background, and description of the ICD classification. The following description includes only those features of immediate relevance to the use of ICD-DA.

The ICD is a systematic classification of diseases, subject to agreement by governments. It is widely used for national mortality and morbidity statistics, and is revised periodically. The Tenth Revision — ICD-10 — came into effect from January 1993; it consists of three separate volumes. Volume 1 includes an explanatory text and a tabular, alphanumeric presentation of the classification. Volume 2 is the instruction manual, which provides coding guidance and general advice on the use of the classification. Volume 3 is a detailed alphabetical index of all diseases and conditions covered by the classification. The taxonomic philosophy of the ICD is necessarily somewhat eclectic: because of differing national views on disease classification and terminology, no strictly systematic classification is entirely practicable.

Volume 1 of ICD-10 is arranged in 21 main sections, or chapters, and this arrangement has been followed for ICD-DA. It also contains a coded nomenclature of the morphology of neoplasms, an extract of which is included in ICD-DA. Not every condition is allotted an individual rubric or number, but there is a category to which every condition can be referred; this has been achieved by the method of selective grouping. The principles for determining which

2

conditions should be assigned to discrete categories are based on frequency, importance, and clarity of characterization of the conditions.

In the alphanumeric system of codes that has been adopted, the detailed categories of the classification are designated by a letter and two numbers. In many instances, the first two characters of the three-character code designate important or summary groups that are significant. The third character divides each summary group into categories that represent either specific disease entities or a classification of diseases or conditions according to some significant axis, such as anatomical site. The three-character categories have not been numbered consecutively: codes have been omitted from the order sequence to preserve the summary character of the first two characters wherever it is meaningful. No additional three-character categories may be introduced into the classification, except when the list is revised by international agreement. Use of a fourth character in the classification allows for more comprehensive studies of the causes of illness and disability.

Efforts have been made to show most of the diagnostic terms given in standard or official nomenclatures, as well as terms commonly used in different countries; these are collectively referred to as "inclusion terms". Where there is any significant risk of a condition being wrongly classified, cross-reference to relevant categories is achieved by means of "exclusion terms". The last two codes at the four-character level (.8 and .9) very often carry the connotation "other" and "unspecified" respectively. The abbreviation "NOS" is attached to many inclusion terms; it stands for "not otherwise specified" and is virtually the equivalent of "unspecified" and "unqualified".

Overall, the arrangement of ICD-10 differs little from that of ICD-9, although there is much additional detail. Certain innovations of ICD-10 are detailed on pages 13–15 of Volume 1.

ICD-DA

Like ICD-10, ICD-DA has a tabular section and a comprehensive alphabetical index. Liberal use has been made of inclusion and exclusion terms in the tabular section to afford users as much assistance as possible in finding the correct category for any condition diagnosed.

Coding system of ICD-DA

Each main code heading in the ICD-DA is an ICD code at the three-character level. Titles for each of these codes and for code groups and main sections remain exactly the same as those given in ICD-10.

However, much of ICD-DA is based on five-character codes related to ICD three- and four-character codes in the following way: the first three or four characters of any ICD-DA code are those of ICD-10; where a fifth character is used it is exclusive to ICD-DA. Where a five-character ICD-DA code relates to a three-character ICD-10 category that has no fourth character subdivisions, a dummy character "X" is used as the fourth character in ICD-DA. In a few instances, a fourth character exists in ICD-10 but is irrelevant to ICD-DA; in these cases it is replaced by the dummy fourth character "V". The fifth character identifies ICD-DA subdivisions of the ICD category; where the ICD-DA identifies a complete ICD category without further subdivisions, the dummy "X" is used as the fifth character. The coding system may be summarized as follows:

Character

1	A–Z	
2	0–9	ICD-10 three-character category
3	0–9	
4	0–9	ICD-10 fourth character
	X	ICD-10 fourth character does not exist
	V	ICD-10 fourth character exists but is not used in ICD-DA
5	0–9	ICD-DA fifth character
	X	ICD-DA fifth character does not exist

Use of the V code enables summaries to be made of oral manifestations of general disease categories. They would not be added to national returns to avoid duplication. The term "oral manifestations" is used in the broadest sense, referring both to conditions that may be observed on clinical inspection, e.g. oral manifestations of zoster (B02.8X), and to conditions not readily observed, e.g. oral manifestations of Albright's syndrome (Q78.1X) affecting the jaws.

Neoplasm section

The section on neoplasms, both malignant and benign, is primarily, and as far as possible, classified according to topography. Similarly, every effort has been made to make the malignant and benign classifications parallel and to distinguish between neoplasms and hyperplasias that are reactive or inflammatory.

4

Extracts from the International Histological Classification of Tumours have been included as annexes to ICD-DA. Those of special interest in the field of oral health are concerned with odontogenic tumours[1] and salivary gland tumours[2] and appear in Annexes 1 and 2 respectively.

For morphological coding of neoplasms, which is not provided by the ICD-DA proper, an extract of the relevant part of the morphology (M) code of the ICD-O[3] is given on pages 132–143.

Recommended use of ICD-DA

ICD-DA may be used at national, regional, institutional, or individual practice level. The recommended procedure is as follows:

1. All diagnoses must be recorded at the appropriate level, i.e. as three-, four-, or five-character codes.

   Pretesting has shown that it is extremely rare to have more than 12 diagnoses for any one patient.

2. The most effective way to introduce and maintain ICD-DA recording is probably office coding of written or electronically recorded diagnoses, rather than direct entry of ICD-DA numbers in clinical records at the time of examination. One clerical assistant, familiar with ICD-DA, could code each day's diagnoses for a number of examiners with a high level of consistency. An example of a form suitable for ICD-DA recording and for annual summary (mostly on the basis of number of cases per population) for national and international use is shown on the next page. Those using ICD-DA will probably find it most convenient to design their own forms, make local arrangements for computer summaries, and keep WHO in Geneva informed of annual results. In case of difficulty, the Oral Health unit of WHO[4] may be able to assist in designing computer summary forms tailored to the needs of a particular institution or country and in performing the annual summaries.

---

[1] Kramer IRH, Pindborg JJ, Shear M. *Histological typing of odontogenic tumours*, 2nd ed. Berlin, Springer-Verlag, 1992.

[2] Seifert G. *Histological typing of salivary gland tumours*, 2nd ed. Berlin, Springer-Verlag, 1991.

[3] *International Classification of Diseases for Oncology, 2nd ed.* Geneva, World Health Organization, 1990.

[4] Oral Health, World Health Organization, 1211 Geneva 27, Switzerland.

Adaptation of existing record systems may be more appropriate for some national systems than introduction of the type of form shown below, but whatever provision is made for use of ICD-DA, allowance should be made for further subdivision resulting from periodic revisions of the ICD and ICD-DA.

3. Until users are familiar with the classification, it is important to consult the index, main headings, and inclusion/exclusion terms before recording a diagnosis.

Example 1

In general, the term "oral mucosa" is applicable to the superficial tissues of the tongue as well as to other soft tissue surfaces of the oral cavity. In many cases, however, there is a separate classification for a set of diseases or conditions depending on whether they occur in the tongue or in other parts of the oral mucosa. Thus K12.11 is geographic stomatitis of oral epithelium, but K14.1 is geographic tongue. Scanning the index under "geographic" should reveal this distinction, but even if the index were to refer only to geographic stomatitis K12.11, the exclusion term would reveal that geographic tongue is K14.1.

SEX M = 0 F = 1 ☐	**ICD–DA CODES**
AGE ☐☐ **YEARS**	1 ☐☐☐☐☐ 9 ☐☐☐☐☐
	2 ☐☐☐☐☐ 10 ☐☐☐☐☐
OPTIONAL CODES	3 ☐☐☐☐☐ 11 ☐☐☐☐☐
	4 ☐☐☐☐☐ 12 ☐☐☐☐☐
OCCUPATION ☐☐	5 ☐☐☐☐☐ 13 ☐☐☐☐☐
ETHNIC GROUP ☐☐	
PATIENT TYPE ☐☐	6 ☐☐☐☐☐ 14 ☐☐☐☐☐
RELIGION ☐☐	7 ☐☐☐☐☐ 15 ☐☐☐☐☐
TYPE OF INSTITUTION ☐☐	8 ☐☐☐☐☐ 16 ☐☐☐☐☐
EXAMINING STAFF ☐☐	

Example 2

The user may rapidly memorize the more important three-character titles such as K05 Gingivitis and periodontal diseases. In a case of, say, acute necrotizing ulcerative gingivitis, consultation of K05.0, Acute gingivitis, before the diagnosis is recorded would show—from the exclusion term— that the correct code for the condition is A69.10.

4. It is usual to reserve .8 and .9 in the first or second decimal place for "other" and "unspecified" conditions. The classification "other" is used for conditions that are specified, but not otherwise classified, e.g. B23.8X HIV disease resulting in other specified conditions—oral manifestations. The classification "unspecified" is used either for an omission in diagnosis, e.g. C00.9, Malignant neoplasm of lip, unspecified, where location on one or other lip has been omitted at examination; or for inability to be specific, e.g. K03.79, Posteruptive colour change of dental hard tissues, unspecified.

5. In coding a case in which the diagnosis is uncertain, the appropriate category must be found to indicate the general nature or site of the lesion, with an "unspecified" diagnosis.

   For example, if it is not established whether a lesion is a radicular cyst or an apical granuloma, the correct code is K04.9, Other and unspecified diseases of the pulp and periapical tissues, because the exact nature of the lesion cannot be specified. It would be incorrect to use two codings—K04.80, Radicular cyst, apical and lateral, and K04.5, Apical granuloma—to indicate the uncertainty.

   Similarly, if a patient has mucosal lesions that might be due to erythema multiforme, lichen planus, or mucous membrane pemphigoid, and the diagnosis is not established with confidence, the correct coding would be K13.79, Lesion of oral mucosa, unspecified; it would be wrong to code all three conditions included in the list of possible diagnoses.

6. In cases where no diagnosis is established, the coding used should indicate the nature, type, or location of the lesion as narrowly as possible. For example, an undiagnosed condition of the lips would be coded K13.09, Disease of lips, unspecified; and a glossitis of undetermined type would be coded K14.09, Glossitis, unspecified.

7. Wherever provision is made for recording oral manifestations of a general disease or condition, the results have no meaning in terms of national statistics for that disease or condition. They do, however, provide an estimate of the frequency of oral manifestations of the disease or condition, a measure that is unlikely to be available consistently elsewhere.

8. Synonyms are provided in parentheses where there is some controversy or in deference to usage, but the title outside parentheses is preferred.

9. Besides multiple topographical involvement, there are times when it is necessary to classify one disease or condition under more than one category. A syndrome (see complete list in index) should be classified by the specific code allotted to it, but certain aspects of the condition, e.g. oral clefts occurring as part of a syndrome, may also need to be classified under other codes.

10. It is essential for the user of ICD-DA to develop a consistent diagnostic system, and certain reference texts will be needed. The Oral Health unit of WHO[1] is prepared to assist by recommending suitable current texts on request.

11. The user should keep in mind the importance of providing feedback to the Oral Health unit of WHO on difficulties encountered in using the ICD-DA, so that improvements can be made.

12. In addition to its application to the collection of data for health statistics, ICD-DA is also being used by oral pathology departments in the context of storage of literature reference cards and collections of slides/transparencies for teaching purposes. Such materials are useful for teaching oral diagnosis, oral medicine, oral pathology, and oral surgery.

---

[1]Oral Health, World Health Organization, 1211 Geneva 27, Switzerland.

ICD-DA tabular list

CHAPTER I

Certain infectious and parasitic diseases

Tuberculosis

A18 **Tuberculosis of other organs**

A18.0 **Tuberculosis of bones and joints**
    A18.00   Jaws
                  Temporomandibular joint

A18.2 **Tuberculous peripheral lymphadenopathy**
    A18.2X   Facial and cervical region

A18.8 **Tuberculosis of other specified organs**
    A18.8X   Mouth

A21 **Tularaemia**

A21.0 **Ulceroglandular tularaemia**
    A21.0X   Oral manifestations

A21.8 **Other forms of tularaemia**
    A21.8X   Oral manifestations

A22 **Anthrax**

A22.8 **Other forms of anthrax**
    A22.8X   Oral manifestations

Certain zoonotic bacterial diseases

A23 **Brucellosis**

A23.0 **Brucellosis due to *Brucella melitensis***
    A23.0X   Oral manifestations

A24 Glanders and melioidosis

A24.3 **Other melioidosis**
A24.3X   Oral manifestations

A28 Other zoonotic bacterial diseases, not elsewhere classified

A28.1 **Cat-scratch disease**
A28.10   Oral manifestations
A28.11   Cervical lymphadenopathy

Other bacterial diseases

A30 Leprosy

A30.VX   Oral manifestations

A31 Infection due to other mycobacteria

A31.8 **Other mycobacterial infections**
A31.80   Oral lesions due to *Mycobacterium intracellulare*
A31.81   Oral lesions due to *Mycobacterium chelonei*
A31.88   Oral lesions due to other and unspecified mycobacteria

A35 Other tetanus

A35.XX   Oral manifestations

A36 Diphtheria

A36.VX   Oral manifestations

A37 Whooping cough

A37.VX   Oral manifestations

A38 Scarlet fever

Excludes: streptococcal gingivostomatitis (K05.00)
A38.XX   Oral manifestations

A39 Meningococcal infection

A39.VX   Oral manifestations

A42 Actinomycosis

A42.2   **Cervicofacial actinomycosis**
A42.2X   Oral manifestations

A43 Nocardiosis

A43.8   **Other forms of nocardiosis**
A43.8X   Oral manifestations

Infections with a predominantly sexual mode of transmission

Excludes: human immunodeficiency virus [HIV] disease (B20–B24)

A50 Congenital syphilis

A50.0   **Early congenital syphilis, symptomatic**
A50.0X   Oral mucous patches

A50.5   **Other late congenital syphilis, symptomatic**
A50.50   Circumoral furrows [Parrot's furrows]
A50.51   Hutchinson's incisors
A50.52   Mulberry molars
A50.58   Other specified oral manifestations
A50.59   Oral manifestation, unspecified

A51 Early syphilis

A51.2   **Primary syphilis of other sites**
A51.2X   Oral manifestations

A51.3   **Secondary syphilis of skin and mucous membranes**
A51.3X   Oral manifestations

A52 Late syphilis

A52.7   **Other symptomatic late syphilis**
A52.70   Gumma of oral tissues
          Excludes: palatal perforation due to syphilis (A52.71)
A52.71   Palatal perforation due to syphilis
A52.72   Syphilitic glossitis
A52.73   Syphilitic osteomyelitis of jaw
A52.78   Other specified oral manifestations
A52.79   Oral manifestation, unspecified

A54 Gonococcal infection

A54.4 Gonococcal infection of musculoskeletal system
A54.4X Gonococcal infection of temporomandibular joint

A54.8 Other gonococcal infections
A54.8X Gonococcal stomatitis

A55 Chlamydial lymphogranuloma (venereum)

A55.XX Oral manifestations

A58 Granuloma inguinale

A58.XX Oral manifestations

Other spirochaetal diseases

A65 Nonvenereal syphilis

Includes: bejel
A65.XX Oral manifestations

A66 Yaws

A66.4 Gummata and ulcers of yaws
A66.4X Oral manifestations

A66.6 Bone and joint lesions of yaws
A66.6X Oral manifestations

A66.7 Other manifestations of yaws
A66.7X Oral manifestations

A69 Other spirochaetal infections

A69.0 Necrotizing ulcerative stomatitis
Cancrum oris
Fusospirochaetal gangrene
Noma
Stomatitis gangrenosa

A69.1 Other Vincent's infections
A69.10 Acute necrotizing ulcerative gingivitis
[fusospirochaetal gingivitis] [Vincent's gingivitis]
A69.11 Vincent's angina

Rickettsioses

A75 **Typhus fever**

A75.VX   Oral manifestations

A77 **Spotted fever [tick-borne rickettsioses]**

A77.VX   Oral manifestations

Arthropod-borne viral fevers and viral haemorrhagic fevers

A93 **Other arthropod-borne viral fevers, not elsewhere classified**

A93.8 **Other specified arthropod-borne viral fevers**
A93.8X   Vesicular stomatitis virus disease [Indiana fever]

Viral infections characterized by skin and mucous membrane lesions

B00 **Herpesviral [herpes simplex] infections**

Excludes: herpangina (B08.5X)

B00.0 **Eczema herpeticum**
B00.0X   Kaposi's varicelliform eruption, oral manifestations

B00.1 **Herpesviral vesicular dermatitis**
B00.10   Herpes simplex facialis
B00.11   Herpes simplex labialis

B00.2 **Herpesviral gingivostomatitis and pharyngotonsillitis**
B00.2X   Herpesviral gingivostomatitis

B00.8 **Other forms of herpesviral infection**
B00.8X   Herpesviral whitlow

B01 **Varicella [chickenpox]**

B01.8 **Varicella with other complications**
B01.8X   Oral manifestations

B02 Zoster [herpes zoster]

Includes: shingles

B02.2 Zoster with other nervous system involvement
B02.20 Postherpetic trigeminal neuralgia
B02.21 Postherpetic neuralgia, other cranial nerves

B02.8 Zoster with other complications
B02.8X Oral manifestations

B03 Smallpox[1]

B05 Measles

B05.8 Measles with other complications
B05.8X Oral manifestations
Koplik's spots

B06 Rubella [German measles]

B06.8 Rubella with other complications
B06.8X Oral manifestations

B07 Viral warts

B07.X0 Oral verruca vulgaris
B07.X1 Oral condyloma acuminatum
B07.X2 Focal epithelial hyperplasia
B07.X8 Other specified oral manifestations
B07.X9 Oral manifestation, unspecified

B08 Other viral infections characterized by skin and mucous membrane lesions, not elsewhere classified

B08.0 Other orthopoxvirus infections
B08.00 Oral manifestations of orf
B08.01 Oral manifestations of vaccinia
B08.08 Oral manifestations of other orthopoxviral infections

---

[1]In 1980 the 33rd World Health Assembly declared that smallpox had been eradicated. The classification is maintained for surveillance purposes.

B08.1   **Molluscum contagiosum**
B08.1X   Oral manifestations

B08.3   **Erythema infectiosum [fifth disease]**
B08.3X   Oral manifestations

B08.4   **Enteroviral vesicular stomatitis with exanthem**
Includes: hand, foot and mouth disease
B08.4X   Enteroviral vesicular stomatitis

B08.5   **Enteroviral vesicular pharyngitis**
Herpangina

B08.8   **Other specified viral infections characterized by skin and mucous membrane lesions**
Includes: epizootic stomatitis
B08.8X   Oral manifestations of foot-and-mouth disease
  Excludes: oral manifestations of hand, foot and mouth disease (B08.4X)

Human immunodeficiency virus [HIV] disease

B20   **Human immunodeficiency virus [HIV] disease resulting in infectious and parasitic diseases**

Excludes: acute HIV infection syndrome (B23.0)

B20.0   **HIV disease resulting in mycobacterial infection**
Includes: HIV disease resulting in tuberculosis
B20.0X   Oral manifestations

B20.1   **HIV disease resulting in other bacterial infections**
B20.1X   Oral manifestations

B20.2   **HIV disease resulting in cytomegaloviral disease**
B20.2X   Oral manifestations

B20.3   **HIV disease resulting in other viral infections**
B20.3X   Oral manifestations

B20.4   **HIV disease resulting in candidiasis**
B20.4X   Oral manifestations

B20.5   **HIV disease resulting in other mycoses**
B20.5X   Oral manifestations

B20.7   **HIV disease resulting in multiple infections**
B20.7X   Oral manifestations

B20.8 **HIV disease resulting in other infectious and parasitic diseases**
B20.8X   Oral manifestations

B20.9 **HIV disease resulting in unspecified infectious or parasitic disease**
Includes: HIV disease resulting in infection NOS
B20.9X   Oral manifestations

B21   Human immunodeficiency virus [HIV] disease resulting in malignant neoplasms

B21.0 **HIV disease resulting in Kaposi's sarcoma**
B21.0X   Oral manifestations

B21.1 **HIV disease resulting in Burkitt's lymphoma**
B21.1X   Oral manifestations

B21.2 **HIV disease resulting in other types of non-Hodgkin's lymphoma**
B21.2X   Oral manifestations

B21.7 **HIV disease resulting in multiple malignant neoplasms**
B21.7X   Oral manifestations

B21.8 **HIV disease resulting in other malignant neoplasms**
B21.8X   Oral manifestations

B21.9 **HIV disease resulting in unspecified malignant neoplasm**
B21.9X   Oral manifestations

B23   Human immunodeficiency virus [HIV] disease resulting in other conditions

B23.0 **Acute HIV infection syndrome**
B23.0X   Oral manifestations

B23.1 **HIV disease resulting in (persistent) generalized lymphadenopathy**
B23.1X   Oral manifestations

B23.8 **HIV disease resulting in other specified conditions**
B23.8X   Oral manifestations

B24 Unspecified human immunodeficiency virus [HIV] disease

Includes: acquired immunodeficiency syndrome [AIDS] NOS
AIDS-related complex [ARC] NOS

B24.XX Oral manifestations

Other viral diseases

B25 Cytomegaloviral disease

B25.8 Other cytomegaloviral diseases
B25.8X Oral manifestations

B26 Mumps

B26.9 Mumps without complication
B26.9X Oral manifestations

B27 Infectious mononucleosis

Includes: glandular fever

B27.8 Other infectious mononucleosis
B27.8X Oral manifestations

Mycoses

Excludes: mycosis fungoides (C84.0)

B35 Dermatophytosis

B35.0 Tinea barbae and tinea capitis
B35.0X Oral manifestations

B37 Candidiasis

Includes: candidosis
moniliasis

B37.0 Candidal stomatitis
B37.00 Acute pseudomembranous candidal stomatitis
B37.01 Acute erythematous (atrophic) candidal stomatitis
B37.02 Chronic hyperplastic candidal stomatitis
Candidal leukoplakia
Multifocal-type chronic hyperplastic candidal stomatitis

19

B37.03	Chronic erythematous (atrophic) candidal stomatitis
	Denture stomatitis due to candidal infection
B37.04	Mucocutaneous candidiasis
B37.05	Oral candidal granuloma
B37.06	Angular cheilitis
B37.08	Other specified oral manifestations
B37.09	Oral manifestation, unspecified
	Oral thrush NOS
	Soor NOS

B38 Coccidioidomycosis

B38.VX   Oral manifestations

B39 Histoplasmosis

B39.VX   Oral manifestations

B40 Blastomycosis

B40.VX   Oral manifestations

B41 Paracoccidioidomycosis

Includes: Brazilian blastomycosis
B41.VX   Oral manifestations

B42 Sporotrichosis

B42.VX   Oral manifestations

B43 Chromomycosis and phaeomycotic abscess

B43.8 **Other forms of chromomycosis**
B43.8X   Oral manifestations

B44 Aspergillosis

B44.8 **Other forms of aspergillosis**
B44.8X   Oral manifestations

B45 Cryptococcosis

B45.8 **Other forms of cryptococcosis**
B45.8X   Oral manifestations

B46 Zygomycosis

B46.5   Mucormycosis, unspecified
B46.5X   Oral manifestations

B47 Mycetoma

B47.VX   Oral manifestations

B48 Other mycoses, not elsewhere classified

B48.1   Rhinosporidiosis
B48.1X   Oral manifestations

B48.3   Geotrichosis
B48.3X   Geotrichum stomatitis

Protozoal diseases

B55 Leishmaniasis

B55.2   Mucocutaneous leishmaniasis
B55.2X   Oral manifestations

B57 Chagas' disease

B57.VX   Oral manifestations

B58 Toxoplasmosis

B58.8   Toxoplasmosis with other organ involvement
B58.8X   Oral manifestations

Helminthiases

B67 Echinococcosis

B67.9   Echinococcosis, other and unspecified
B67.9X   Oral manifestations

B68 Taeniasis

Excludes: cysticercosis (B69. –)
B68.VX   Oral manifestations

B69 Cysticercosis

B69.8 Cysticercosis of other sites
B69.8X Oral manifestations

B74 Filariasis

B74.VX Oral manifestations

B75 Trichinellosis

B75.XX Oral manifestations

B76 Hookworm diseases

B76.VX Oral manifestations

B77 Ascariasis

B77.VX Oral manifestations

B79 Trichuriasis

B79.XX Oral manifestations

B83 Other helminthiases

B83.VX Oral manifestations

Pediculosis, acariasis and other infestations

B87 Myiasis

B87.8 Myiasis of other sites
B87.8X Oral manifestations

CHAPTER II

Neoplasms

Notes

1. Primary, ill-defined, secondary and unspecified sites of malignant neoplasms

Categories C00–C75 and C81–C96 include malignant neoplasms stated or presumed to be primary.

Categories C76–C80 include malignant neoplasms where there is no clear indication of the original site of the cancer or the cancer is stated to be "disseminated", "scattered" or "spread" without mention of the primary site. In both cases the primary site is considered to be unknown.

2. Functional activity

All neoplasms related to the oral cavity are classified in this chapter, whether they are functionally active or not.

3. Morphology

There are a number of major morphological (histological) groups of malignant neoplasms: carcinomas including squamous (cell) and adenocarcinomas; sarcomas; other soft tissue tumours including mesotheliomas; lymphomas (Hodgkin's and non-Hodgkin's); leukaemia; other specified and site-specific types; and unspecified cancers. Cancer is a generic term and may be used for any of the above groups although it is rarely applied to the malignant neoplasms of lymphatic, haematopoietic and related tissue. "Carcinoma" is sometimes used incorrectly as a synonym for "cancer".

In Chapter II neoplasms are classified predominantly by site within broad groupings for behaviour. In a few exceptional cases morphology is indicated in the category and subcategory titles.

For those wishing to identify the histological type of neoplasm, comprehensive separate morphology codes are provided on pages 132–143. These morphology codes are derived from the International Classification of Diseases for Oncology, second edition (ICD-O), which is a dual-axis classification providing independent coding systems for topography and morphology. These codes have six digits: the first four digits identify the histological type; the fifth digit is the behaviour code (malignant primary, malignant secondary (metastatic), in situ, benign, uncertain whether malignant or benign); and the sixth digit is a grading code (differentiation) for solid tumours and is also used as a special code for lymphomas and leukaemias, but is not included in ICD-DA.

The ICD-O behaviour digit /9 is not applicable in the ICD context, since all malignant neoplasms are presumed to be primary (/3) or secondary (/6), according to other information on the medical record.

4. Use of subcategories in Chapter II

Attention is drawn to the special use of subcategory .8 in this chapter (see note 5). Where it has been necessary to provide subcategories for "other", these have generally been designated as subcategory .7.

5. Malignant neoplasms overlapping site boundaries and the use of subcategory .8 (overlapping lesion)

Categories C00–C75 classify primary malignant neoplasms according to their point of origin. Many three-character categories are further divided into named parts or subcategories of the organ in question. A neoplasm that overlaps two or more contiguous sites within a three-character category and whose point of origin cannot be determined should be classified to the subcategory .8 ("overlapping lesion"), unless the combination is specifically indexed elsewhere. For example, carcinoma of the tip and ventral surface of the tongue should be assigned to C02.8, while carcinoma of the tip of the tongue extending to involve the ventral surface should be coded to C02.1 as the point of origin, the tip, is known. "Overlapping" implies that the sites involved are contiguous (next to each other). Numerically consecutive subcategories are frequently anatomically contiguous, but this is not invariably so and the coder may need to consult anatomical texts to determine the topographical relationships.

Sometimes a neoplasm overlaps the boundaries of three-character categories within certain systems. To take care of this the subcategories that have been designated include the following:

C02.8 Overlapping lesion of tongue
C08.8 Overlapping lesion of major salivary glands

C14.8   Overlapping lesion of lip, oral cavity and pharynx
C41.8   Overlapping lesion of bone and auricular cartilage

6.   Malignant neoplasms of ectopic tissue

Malignant neoplasms of ectopic tissue are to be coded to the site mentioned.

7.   Use of the Alphabetical Index in coding neoplasms

In addition to site, morphology and behaviour must also be taken into consideration when coding neoplasms, and reference should always be made first to the Alphabetical Index entry for the morphological description.

The introductory pages of Volume 3 of ICD-10 include general instructions about the correct use of the Alphabetical Index. The specific instructions and examples pertaining to neoplasms in Volume 2 should be consulted to ensure correct use of the categories and subcategories in Chapter II.

8.   Use of the second edition of the International Classification of Diseases for Oncology (ICD-O)

For certain morphological types, Chapter II provides a rather restricted topographical classification, or none at all. The topography codes of ICD-O use, for all neoplasms, essentially the same three- and four-character categories that Chapter II uses for primary malignant neoplasms (C00–C76, C80), thus providing increased specificity of site for other neoplasms (malignant secondary (metastatic), benign, in situ and uncertain or unknown). In addition to the topography and morphology codes, ICD-O also includes a list of tumour-like lesions and conditions.

It is therefore recommended that those interested in identifying both the site and morphology of tumours, e.g. cancer registries, cancer hospitals, pathology departments and other agencies specializing in cancer, use ICD-O.

Malignant neoplasms

Malignant neoplasms of lip, oral cavity and pharynx

C00   Malignant neoplasm of lip

Excludes: skin of lip (C43.0, C44.0)

C00.0 **External upper lip**
C00.0X   Vermilion border (lipstick area) of upper lip

C00.1 **External lower lip**
C00.1X   Vermilion border (lipstick area) of lower lip

C00.2 **External lip, unspecified**
C00.2X   Vermilion border (lipstick area) NOS

C00.3 **Upper lip, inner aspect**
Includes: frenulum
Excludes: sulcus (C06.1)
C00.3X   Labial mucosa

C00.4 **Lower lip, inner aspect**
Includes: frenulum
Excludes: sulcus (C06.1)
C00.4X   Labial mucosa

C00.5 **Lip, unspecified, inner aspect**
C00.5X   Labial mucosa, not specified whether upper
or lower

C00.6 **Commissure of lip**

C00.8 **Overlapping lesion of lip**
[See note 5 on page 24]

C00.9 **Lip, unspecified**
Not specified whether upper or lower lip; location on lip not specified

C01 Malignant neoplasm of base of tongue

Dorsal surface of base of tongue
Posterior third of tongue

C02 Malignant neoplasm of other and unspecified parts of tongue

C02.0 **Dorsal surface of tongue**
C02.0X   Anterior two-thirds of tongue, dorsal surface
Excludes: dorsal surface of base of tongue (C01)

C02.1 **Border of tongue**
C02.10   Tip of tongue
C02.11   Lateral border of tongue

C02.2 **Ventral surface of tongue**
C02.2X   Anterior two-thirds of tongue, ventral surface
Lingual frenulum

C02.3 **Anterior two thirds of tongue, part unspecified**

C02.4 **Lingual tonsil**
Excludes: tonsil NOS (C09.9)

C02.8 **Overlapping lesion of tongue**
[See note 5 on page 24]

C02.9 **Tongue, unspecified**

C03   Malignant neoplasm of gum

Includes: alveolar (ridge) mucosa
gingiva
Excludes: malignant odontogenic neoplasms (C41.0–C41.1)

C03.0 **Upper gum**
C03.0X   Maxilla, gingiva and alveolar ridge mucosa
Excludes: maxillary tuberosity (C06.20)

C03.1 **Lower gum**
C03.1X   Mandible, gingiva and alveolar ridge mucosa
Excludes: mandibular retromolar area (C06.21)

C03.9 **Gum, unspecified**
C03.9X   Gingiva and alveolar ridge, jaw unspecified

C04   Malignant neoplasm of floor of mouth

Excludes: ventral surface of tongue (C02.2X)

C04.0 **Anterior floor of mouth**

C04.1 **Lateral floor of mouth**

C04.8 **Overlapping lesion of floor of mouth**
[See note 5 on page 24]

C04.9 **Floor of mouth, unspecified**

C05   Malignant neoplasm of palate

C05.0 **Hard palate**

C05.1 **Soft palate**
Excludes: nasopharyngeal surface of soft palate (C11.3X)

C05.2 **Uvula**

C05.8 **Overlapping lesion**
[See note 5 on page 24]

C05.9   Palate, unspecified

C06   Malignant neoplasm of other and unspecified parts of mouth

Excludes: mucosa of lips (C00.–)

C06.0   Buccal mucosa
Excludes: labial commissure (C00.6)
sulcus (C06.1)

C06.1   Vestibule of mouth
C06.10   Upper labial sulcus
C06.11   Upper buccal sulcus
C06.12   Lower labial sulcus
C06.13   Lower buccal sulcus
C06.14   Upper sulcus, unspecified
C06.15   Lower sulcus, unspecified
C06.19   Vestibule of mouth, unspecified

C06.2   Retromolar area
C06.20   Maxillary tuberosity
C06.21   Mandibular retromolar area
C06.29   Retromolar area, unspecified

C06.8   Overlapping lesion of other and unspecified parts of mouth
[See note 5 on page 24]

C06.9   Mouth, unspecified
Oral cavity NOS

C07   Malignant neoplasm of parotid gland

C08   Malignant neoplasm of other and unspecified major salivary glands

Excludes: malignant neoplasms of specified minor salivary glands which are classified according to their anatomical location
malignant neoplasms of minor salivary glands NOS (C06.9)
parotid gland (C07)

C08.0   Submandibular gland
Submaxillary gland

C08.1   Sublingual gland

C08.8 **Overlapping lesion of major salivary glands**
[See note 5 on page 24]

C08.9 **Major salivary gland, unspecified**
Salivary gland (major) NOS

C09 Malignant neoplasm of tonsil

Excludes: lingual tonsil (C02.4)
pharyngeal tonsil (C11.1)

C09.0 **Tonsillar fossa**

C09.1 **Tonsillar pillar**

C09.8 **Overlapping lesion of tonsil**
[See note 5 on page 24]

C09.9 **Tonsil, unspecified**
Palatine tonsil

C10 Malignant neoplasm of oropharynx

Excludes: tonsil (C09.–)

C10.0 **Vallecula**

C10.2 **Lateral wall of oropharynx**

C10.3 **Posterior wall of oropharynx**

C10.4 **Branchial cleft**
Branchial cyst [site of neoplasm]

C10.8 **Overlapping lesion of oropharynx**
[See note 5 on page 24]

C10.9 **Oropharynx, unspecified**

C11 Malignant neoplasm of nasopharynx

C11.1 **Posterior wall of nasopharynx**

C11.3 **Anterior wall of nasopharynx**
C11.3X   Nasopharyngeal surface of soft palate

C14 Malignant neoplasm of other and ill-defined sites in the lip, oral cavity and pharynx

Excludes: oral cavity NOS (C06.9)

C14.8 **Overlapping lesion of lip, oral cavity and pharynx**
[See note 5 on page 24]
Malignant neoplasm of lip, oral cavity and pharynx whose point of origin cannot be classified to any one of the categories C00–C14.2 included in this classification

Malignant neoplasms of respiratory and intrathoracic organs

C30 Malignant neoplasm of nasal cavity and middle ear

C30.0 **Nasal cavity**
Excludes: nasal bone (C41.0)
skin of nose (C43.3, C44.3)

C31 Malignant neoplasm of accessory sinuses

C31.0 **Maxillary sinus**

C31.1 **Ethmoidal sinus**

C31.2 **Frontal sinus**

C31.3 **Sphenoidal sinus**

C31.8 **Overlapping lesion of accessory sinuses**
[See note 5 on page 24]

C31.9 **Accessory sinus, unspecified**

Malignant neoplasms of bone and articular cartilage

C41 Malignant neoplasm of bone and articular cartilage of other and unspecified sites

C41.0 **Bones of skull and face**
Excludes: carcinoma, any type other than odontogenic or intra-osseous salivary gland tumour (C03.0, C31.1, C41.1)
    C41.00 Maxilla, sarcoma
          Excludes: odontogenic sarcoma (C41.01)
    C41.01 Maxilla, malignant odontogenic tumour
          Carcinoma arising in odontogenic cyst
    C41.02 Maxilla, malignant intraosseous salivary gland tumour
    C41.09 Maxilla, unspecified

C41.1 Mandible
Includes: jaw NOS
Excludes: carcinoma, any type other than odontogenic or intra-
osseous salivary gland tumour (C03.1, C31.9, C41.0)

C41.10 Sarcoma
Excludes: odontogenic sarcoma (C41.11)

C41.11 Malignant odontogenic tumour
Carcinoma arising in odontogenic cyst

C41.12 Malignant intraosseous salivary gland tumour

C41.19 Mandible, unspecified

C41.8 Overlapping lesion of bone and articular cartilage
[See note 5 on page 24]
Malignant neoplasm of bone and articular cartilage whose point of
origin cannot be classified to any one of the categories C40–C41.4
included in this classification

Melanoma and other malignant neoplasms of skin

C43 Malignant melanoma of skin

C43.0 Malignant melanoma of lip
Excludes: vermilion border of lip (C00.0–C00.2)
labial mucosa (C00.3–C00.5)

C43.3 Malignant melanoma of other and unspecified parts of face

C43.8 Overlapping malignant melanoma of skin
[See note 5 on page 24]

C44 Other malignant neoplasms of skin

Excludes: Kaposi's sarcoma (C46.–)
malignant melanoma of skin (C43.–)

C44.0 Skin of lip
Excludes: vermilion border (C00.0–C00.2)
labial mucosa (C00.3–C00.5)

C44.3 Skin of other and unspecified parts of face

C44.8 Overlapping lesion of skin
[See note 5 on page 24]

Malignant neoplasms of mesothelial and soft tissue

C46 Kaposi's sarcoma

C46.0 **Kaposi's sarcoma of skin**
C46.0X   Facial skin

C46.1 **Kaposi's sarcoma of soft tissue**
C46.1X   Oral soft tissues
Excludes: palate (C46.2)

C46.2 **Kaposi's sarcoma of palate**

C46.3 **Kaposi's sarcoma of lymph nodes**
C46.3X   Cervicofacial nodes

C47 Malignant neoplasm of peripheral nerves and autonomic nervous system

C47.0 **Peripheral nerves of head, face and neck**
Excludes: cranial nerves (C72.–)

C49 Malignant neoplasm of other connective and soft tissue

C49.0 **Connective and soft tissue of head, face and neck**

Malignant neoplasms of eye, brain and other parts of central nervous system

C72 Malignant neoplasm of spinal cord, cranial nerves and other parts of central nervous system

C72.5 **Other and unspecified cranial nerves**
Includes: facial
hypoglossal
trigeminal
C72.5X   Oral manifestations

Malignant neoplasms of ill-defined, secondary and unspecified sites

C76   Malignant neoplasm of other and ill-defined sites

C76.0   **Head, face and neck**
Head, face and neck NOS

C77   Secondary and unspecified malignant neoplasm of lymph nodes

Excludes: malignant neoplasm of lymph nodes, specified as primary (C81–C88, C96.–)

C77.0   **Lymph nodes of head, face and neck**

C79   Secondary malignant neoplasm of other sites

C79.2   **Secondary malignant neoplasm of skin**
C79.2X   Face
          Lips

C79.5   **Secondary malignant neoplasm of bone and bone marrow**
C79.50   Maxilla
C79.51   Mandible
          Condyle
C79.58   Other specified facial bones
C79.59   Facial bone, unspecified

C79.8   **Secondary malignant neoplasm of other specified sites**
C79.8X   Oral tissues
          Tongue

Malignant neoplasms of lymphoid, haematopoietic and related tissue

Note: A detailed classification of these neoplasms (C81–C96) may be found in ICD-10.

Excludes: secondary and unspecified neoplasm of lymph nodes (C77.–)

C81   Hodgkin's disease

C81.VX   Oral manifestations

C82   Follicular [nodular] non-Hodgkin's lymphoma

C82.VX   Oral manifestations

C83   Diffuse non-Hodgkin's lymphoma

Includes: morphology codes M9593, M9595, M967–M968 with behaviour code /3

C83.3   Large cell (diffuse)
Includes: reticulum cell sarcoma
C83.3X   Oral manifestations

C83.7   Burkitt's tumour
C83.7X   Oral manifestations

C84   Peripheral and cutaneous T-cell lymphomas

C84.0   Mycosis fungoides
C84.0X   Oral manifestations

C85   Other and unspecified types of non-Hodgkin's lymphoma

Includes: morphology codes M9590–M9592, M9594, M971 with behaviour code /3

C85.0   Lymphosarcoma
C85.0X   Oral manifestations

C88   Malignant immunoproliferative diseases

Includes: morphology code M976 with behaviour code /3

C88.0   Waldenström's macroglobulinaemia
C88.0X   Oral manifestations

C90   Multiple myeloma and malignant plasma cell neoplasms

Includes: morphology code M973 with behaviour code /3

C90.0   Multiple myeloma
Excludes: solitary myeloma (C90.2)
C90.0X   Oral manifestations

C90.2   **Plasmacytoma, extramedullary**
Includes: malignant plasma cell tumour NOS
plasmacytoma NOS
solitary myeloma
C90.2X   Oral manifestations

C91   **Lymphoid leukaemia**

C91.VX   Oral manifestations

C92   **Myeloid leukaemia**

C92.VX   Oral manifestations
Chloroma

C93   **Monocytic leukaemia**

C93.VX   Oral manifestations

C94   **Other leukaemias of specified cell type**

C94.0   **Acute erythraemia and erythroleukaemia**
C94.0X   Oral manifestations

C95   **Leukaemia of unspecified cell type**

Includes: morphology code M980 with behaviour code /3
C95.VX   Oral manifestations

C96   **Other and unspecified malignant neoplasms of lymphoid, haematopoietic and related tissue**

Includes: morphology codes M972, M974 with behaviour code /3

C96.0   **Letterer–Siwe disease**
C96.0X   Oral manifestations

Malignant neoplasms of independent (primary) multiple sites

C97   **Malignant neoplasms of independent (primary) multiple sites**

C97.XX   Primary malignant neoplasm of mouth with concurrent primary malignant neoplasm of other site(s)

In situ neoplasms

Note: Many in situ neoplasms are regarded as being located within a continuum of morphological change between dysplasia and invasive cancer. For example, for cervical intraepithelial neoplasia (CIN) three grades are recognized, the third of which (CIN III) includes both severe dysplasia and carcinoma in situ. This system of grading has been extended to other organs, e.g. oral mucosa. Descriptions of grade III intraepithelial neoplasia, with or without mention of severe dysplasia, are assigned to this section; grades I and II are classified as dysplasia of the organ system involved and should be coded to the relevant body system chapter.

Includes: Bowen's disease
erythroplakia
erythroplasia
morphology codes with behaviour code /2

D00 Carcinoma in situ of oral cavity, oesophagus and stomach

Excludes: melanoma in situ (D03.–)

D00.0 Lip, oral cavity and pharynx
Excludes: skin of lip (D03.0, D04.0)
D00.00 Labial mucosa and vermilion border
D00.01 Buccal mucosa
D00.02 Gingiva and edentulous alveolar ridge
D00.03 Palate
D00.04 Floor of mouth
D00.05 Ventral surface of tongue
D00.06 Tongue other than ventral surface
D00.07 Oropharynx
D00.08 Other specified carcinoma in situ of oral cavity, oesophagus and stomach
D00.09 Unspecified carcinoma in situ of oral cavity, oesophagus and stomach

D02 Carcinoma in situ of middle ear and respiratory system

Excludes: melanoma in situ (D03.–)

D02.3 Other parts of respiratory system
D02.3X Nasal cavity and accessory sinuses

D03   Melanoma in situ

Includes: morphology codes M872–M879 with behaviour code /2

D03.0   **Melanoma in situ of lip**
D03.0X   Labial mucosa and vermilion border

D03.3   **Melanoma in situ of other and unspecified parts of face**
D03.30   Skin of lip
D03.31   Other facial skin

D03.8   **Melanoma in situ of other sites**
D03.8X   Melanoma in situ of oral mucosa
         Excludes: melanoma in situ, labial mucosa (D03.0X)

D04   Carcinoma in situ of skin

Excludes: melanoma in situ (D03.–)

D04.0   **Skin of lip**
Excludes: vermilion border of lip (D00.0)

D04.3   **Skin of other and unspecified parts of face**

Benign neoplasms

Includes: morphology codes with behaviour code /0

D10   Benign neoplasm of mouth and pharynx

D10.0   **Lip**
Includes: labial commissure (D10.3)
Excludes: skin of lip (D22.0, D23.0)
         benign neoplasm of minor salivary glands
D10.00   Upper lip, vermilion border
D10.01   Upper lip, labial mucosa
D10.02   Upper lip, vermilion border with mucosa
D10.03   Lower lip, vermilion border
D10.04   Lower lip, labial mucosa
D10.05   Lower lip, vermilion border with mucosa
D10.06   Both lips, vermilion border
D10.07   Both lips, labial mucosa
D10.08   Both lips, vermilion border with mucosa
D10.09   Lip, unspecified

D10.1   **Tongue**
Includes: benign neoplasm of minor salivary glands
D10.10   Base of tongue (posterior to terminal sulcus)

D10.11　Dorsal surface of tongue
D10.12　Borders and tip of tongue
D10.13　Ventral surface of tongue
D10.14　Lingual tonsil
D10.19　Tongue, unspecified

D10.2　Floor of mouth

D10.3　Other and unspecified parts of mouth
Includes: minor salivary gland NOS
Excludes: benign odontogenic neoplasms (D16.4–D16.5)
　　　　　mucosa of lip (D10.0)
　　　　　nasopharyngeal surface of soft palate (D10.6)
D10.30　Buccal mucosa
D10.31　Buccal mucosal commissure
D10.32　Buccal sulcus
D10.33　Gingiva and edentulous alveolar ridge
　　　　Congenital epulis
　　　　Excludes: fibrous epulis (K06.82)
　　　　　　　　giant cell granuloma, peripheral (K06.81)
　　　　　　　　pregnancy granuloma (O26.8)
D10.34　Hard palate
　　　　Junction of hard and soft palate
D10.35　Soft palate
D10.36　Uvula
D10.37　Retromolar area
D10.38　Tuberosity
D10.39　Mouth, unspecified

D10.4　Tonsil
Excludes: lingual tonsil (D10.1)
　　　　　tonsillar (faucial) pillars and tonsillar fossa (D10.5)

D10.5　Other parts of oropharynx
Tonsillar (faucial) pillars and tonsillar fossa

D10.6　Nasopharynx

D10.7　Hypopharynx

D10.9　Pharynx, unspecified

D11　Benign neoplasm of major salivary glands

Excludes: benign neoplasms of specified minor salivary glands which
　　　　　are classified according to their anatomical location
　　　　　benign neoplasms of minor salivary glands NOS (D10.3)

D11.0　Parotid gland

D11.7 **Other major salivary glands**
D11.70 Submandibular gland
   Submaxillary gland
D11.71 Sublingual gland

D11.9 **Major salivary gland, unspecified**

D14 Benign neoplasm of middle ear and respiratory system

D14.0 **Middle ear, nasal cavity and accessory sinuses**
D14.0X Nasal and accessory sinuses
   Maxillary sinus

D16 Benign neoplasm of bone and articular cartilage

Includes: odontogenic tissues
Excludes: cherubism (K10.80)
   exostosis of jaw (K10.88)
   fibrous dysplasia of jaw (K10.83)
   giant cell granuloma (K10.1)
   tori of jaw (K10.00)

D16.4 **Bones of skull and face**
D16.40 Maxilla, bone and cartilage
D16.41 Maxilla, odontogenic tissues

D16.5 **Lower jaw bone**
D16.50 Mandible, bone and cartilage
D16.51 Mandible, odontogenic tissues

D16.9 **Bone and articular cartilage, unspecified**
D16.90 Bone and cartilage
D16.91 Odontogenic tissues

D17 Benign lipomatous neoplasm

Includes: morphology codes M885–M888 with behaviour code /0

D17.0 **Benign lipomatous neoplasm of skin and subcutaneous tissue of head, face and neck**

D18 Haemangioma and lymphangioma, any site

Includes: morphology codes M912–M917 with behaviour code /0

D18.0 **Haemangioma, any site**
D18.0X Oral manifestations

D18.1 **Lymphangioma, any site**
D18.1X   Oral manifestations

D21 **Other benign neoplasms of connective and other soft tissue**

D21.0 **Connective and other soft tissue of head, face and neck**
Benign tumours of blood vessels other than haemangioma and
  glomus tumour
Leiomyoma
Rhabdomyoma
Excludes: benign neoplasms of cranial nerves (D33.3)

D22 **Melanocytic naevi**

Includes: morphology codes M872–M879 with behaviour code /0
            naevus:
            • NOS
            • blue
            • hairy
            • pigmented

D22.0 **Melanocytic naevi of lip**
Excludes: vermilion border of lip (D10.0)

D22.3 **Melanocytic naevi of other and unspecified parts of face**

D23 **Other benign neoplasms of skin**

Includes: benign neoplasm of:
            • hair follicles
            • sebaceous glands
            • sweat glands

D23.0 **Skin of lip**
Excludes: vermilion border (D10.0)

D23.3 **Skin of other and unspecified parts of face**

D33 **Benign neoplasm of brain and other parts of central nervous system**

D33.3 **Cranial nerves**

D36 **Benign neoplasm of other and unspecified sites**

D36.0 **Lymph nodes**
D36.0X   Head and neck

D36.1   Peripheral nerves and autonomic nervous system
D36.1X   Head and neck

Neoplasms of uncertain or unknown behaviour

D37   Neoplasm of uncertain or unknown behaviour of oral cavity and digestive organs

D37.0   Lip, oral cavity and pharynx
D37.00   Major salivary glands
D37.01   Minor salivary glands
D37.08   Other specified oral locations
D37.09   Oral location, unspecified

D38   Neoplasm of uncertain or unknown behaviour of middle ear and respiratory and intrathoracic organs

D38.5   Other respiratory organs
D38.50   Maxillary sinus
D38.51   Other sinuses

D43   Neoplasm of uncertain or unknown behaviour of brain and central nervous system

Excludes: peripheral nerves and autonomic nervous system (D48.2)

D43.3   Cranial nerves

D45   Polycythaemia vera

Includes: morphology code M9950 with behaviour code /1
D45.XX   Oral manifestations

D47   Other neoplasms of uncertain or unknown behaviour of lymphoid, haematopoietic and related tissue

Includes: morphology codes M974, M976, M996–M997 with
behaviour code /1

D47.0   Histiocytic and mast cell tumours of uncertain and unknown behaviour
D47.0X   Oral manifestations

D48 Neoplasm of uncertain or unknown behaviour of other and unspecified sites

Excludes: neurofibromatosis (nonmalignant) (Q85.0)

D48.0 **Bone and articular cartilage**
D48.0X   Oral manifestations

D48.1 **Connective and other soft tissue**
D48.1X   Oral manifestations

D48.2 **Peripheral nerves and autonomic nervous system**
D48.2X   Oral manifestations

D48.5 **Skin**
Excludes: vermilion border of lip (D37.0)
D48.5X   Oral manifestations

D48.9 **Neoplasm of uncertain or unknown behaviour, unspecified**
Includes: "growth" NOS
neoplasm NOS
new growth NOS
tumour NOS
D48.9X   Oral manifestations

Diseases of the blood and blood-forming organs and certain disorders involving the immune mechanism

Nutritional anaemias

D50 **Iron deficiency anaemia**

D50.0 **Iron deficiency anaemia secondary to blood loss (chronic)**
D50.0X   Oral manifestations

D50.1 **Sideropenic dysphagia**
Includes: Kelly–Paterson syndrome
Plummer–Vinson syndrome
D50.1X   Oral manifestations

D50.8 **Other iron deficiency anaemias**
D50.8X   Oral manifestations

D50.9 **Iron deficiency anaemia, unspecified**
D50.9X   Oral manifestations

D51 **Vitamin B$_{12}$ deficiency anaemia**

D51.VX   Oral manifestations

D52 **Folate deficiency anaemia**

D52.VX   Oral manifestations

D53 **Other nutritional anaemias**

D53.VX   Oral manifestations

Haemolytic anaemias

D55 **Anaemia due to enzyme disorders**

D55.VX   Oral manifestations

D56 **Thalassaemia**

Includes: anaemia:
• Cooley's
• Mediterranean
D56.VX   Oral manifestations

D57 **Sickle-cell disorders**

D57.VX   Oral manifestations

D58 **Other hereditary haemolytic anaemias**

D58.VX   Oral manifestations

D59 **Acquired haemolytic anaemia**

D59.VX   Oral manifestations

Aplastic and other anaemias

D61 **Other aplastic anaemias**

D61.VX   Oral manifestations

Coagulation defects, purpura and other haemorrhagic conditions

D65 **Disseminated intravascular coagulation [defibrination syndrome]**

D65.XX   Oral manifestations

D66 **Hereditary factor VIII deficiency**

D66.XX   Oral manifestations

D67 **Hereditary factor IX deficiency**

D67.XX   Oral manifestations

D68 **Other coagulation defects**

D68.0 **Von Willebrand's disease**
D68.0X   Oral manifestations

D68.1 **Hereditary factor XI deficiency**
D68.1X   Oral manifestations

D68.2 **Hereditary deficiency of other clotting factors**
D68.2X   Oral manifestations

D68.3 **Haemorrhagic disorder due to circulating anticoagulants**
D68.3X   Oral manifestations

D68.4 **Acquired coagulation factor deficiency**
D68.4X   Oral manifestations

D68.8 **Other specified coagulation defects**
D68.8X   Oral manifestations

D68.9 **Coagulation defect, unspecified**
D68.9X   Oral manifestations

D69   Purpura and other haemorrhagic conditions

D69.0 **Allergic purpura**
D69.0X   Oral manifestations

D69.1 **Qualitative platelet defects**
D69.1X   Oral manifestations

D69.3 **Idiopathic thrombocytopenic purpura**
D69.3X   Oral manifestations

D69.6 **Thrombocytopenia, unspecified**
D69.6X   Oral manifestations

D69.9 **Haemorrhagic condition, unspecified**
D69.9X   Oral manifestations

Other diseases of blood and blood-forming organs

D70   Agranulocytosis

D70.X0   Agranulocytic angina, oral manifestations
D70.X1   Cyclic (periodic) neutropenia, oral manifestations
D70.X2   Drug-induced neutropenia, oral manifestations
D70.X3   Neutropenia NOS, oral manifestations

D71   Functional disorders of polymorphonuclear neutrophils

Includes: chronic (childhood) granulomatous disease
D71.XX   Oral manifestations

D72 Other disorders of white blood cells

D72.8 Other specified disorders of white blood cells
D72.8X Oral manifestations

D72.9 Disorder of white blood cells, unspecified
D72.9X Oral manifestations

D75 Other diseases of blood and blood-forming organs

Includes: polycythaemia
Excludes: polycythaemia vera (D45)
D75.VX Oral manifestations

D76 Certain diseases involving lymphoreticular tissue and reticulohistiocytic system

Excludes: Letterer–Siwe disease

D76.0 Langerhans' cell histiocytosis, not elsewhere classified
Includes: histiocytosis X (chronic)
D76.00 Eosinophilic granuloma, oral manifestations
Excludes: eosinophilic granuloma of oral mucosa (K13.41)
D76.01 Hand–Schüller–Christian disease, oral manifestations

D76.3 Other histiocytosis syndromes
Includes: xanthogranuloma
D76.3X Oral manifestations

Certain disorders involving the immune mechanism

Includes: defects in the complement system
immunodeficiency disorders, except human immunodeficiency
virus [HIV] disease
sarcoidosis
Excludes: functional disorders of polymorphonuclear neutrophils (D71)
human immunodeficiency virus [HIV] disease (B20–B24)

D80 Immunodeficiency with predominantly antibody defects

Includes: hypogammaglobulinaemia
agammaglobulinaemia
D80.VX Oral manifestations

D82 Immunodeficiency associated with other major defects

D82.0 **Wiskott–Aldrich syndrome**
D82.0X   Oral manifestations

D82.1 **Di George's syndrome**
D82.1X   Oral manifestations

D86 Sarcoidosis

D86.8 **Sarcoidosis of other and combined sites**
Includes: uveoparotid fever [Heerfordt]
D86.8X   Oral manifestations

D89 Other disorders involving the immune mechanism, not elsewhere classified

D89.0 **Polyclonal hypergammaglobulinaemia**
Includes: benign hypergammaglobulinaemic purpura
D89.0X   Oral manifestations

CHAPTER IV

Endocrine, nutritional and metabolic diseases

Disorders of the thyroid gland

E07   Other disorders of thyroid

E07.9   **Disorder of thyroid, unspecified**
        E07.9X   Oral manifestations

Note: If a more detailed specification of thyroid disorders is required, refer
to ICD-10, E00–E07.

Diabetes mellitus

E14   Unspecified diabetes mellitus

        E14.XX   Oral manifestations

Note: If a more detailed specification of diabetes mellitus is required, refer to
ICD-10, E10–E14.

Disorders of other endocrine glands

E20   Hypoparathyroidism

        E20.VX   Oral manifestations
                      Pseudohypoparathyroidism

E21   Hyperparathyroidism and other disorders of parathyroid gland

E21.0   **Primary hyperparathyroidism**
        E21.0X   Oral manifestations

E21.1   **Secondary hyperparathyroidism, not elsewhere classified**
        E21.1X   Oral manifestations

E21.3 Hyperparathyroidism, unspecified
E21.3X   Oral manifestations

E22 Hyperfunction of pituitary gland

E22.0 Acromegaly and pituitary gigantism
E22.00   Oral manifestations of acromegaly
E22.01   Oral manifestations of gigantism

E23 Hypofunction and other disorders of pituitary gland

E23.0 Hypopituitarism
E23.00   Oral manifestations of Simmonds' disease
E23.01   Oral manifestations of idiopathic growth hormone
         deficiency

E23.6 Other disorders of pituitary gland
E23.60   Oral manifestations of adiposogenital dystrophy
E23.61   Oral manifestations of Fröhlich's syndrome

E27 Other disorders of adrenal gland

E27.1 Primary adrenocortical insufficiency
E27.1X   Oral manifestations of Addison's disease

E31 Polyglandular dysfunction

E31.VX Oral manifestations

E34 Other endocrine disorders

E34.8 Other specified endocrine disorders
E34.8X   Oral manifestations of progeria

Malnutrition

E40 Kwashiorkor

E40.XX   Oral manifestations

E41 Nutritional marasmus

E41.XX   Oral manifestations

Other nutritional deficiencies

E50 Vitamin A deficiency

E50.8 **Other manifestations of vitamin A deficiency**
E50.8X   Oral manifestations

E51 Thiamine deficiency

E51.1 **Beriberi**
E51.1X   Oral manifestations

E52 Niacin deficiency [pellagra]

E52.XX   Oral manifestations

E53 Deficiency of other B group vitamins

E53.0 **Riboflavin deficiency**
E53.0X   Oral manifestations

E53.8 **Deficiency of other specified B group vitamins**
E53.8X   Oral manifestations

E54 Ascorbic acid deficiency

E54.XX   Oral manifestations

E55 Vitamin D deficiency

Excludes: adult osteomalacia (M83.–)
osteoporosis (M80–M81)

E55.0 **Rickets, active**
E55.0X   Oral manifestations

E56 Other vitamin deficiencies

E56.1 **Deficiency of vitamin K**
E56.1X   Oral manifestations

E56.8 **Deficiency of other vitamins**
E56.8X   Oral manifestations

E56.9 **Vitamin deficiency, unspecified**
E56.9X   Oral manifestations

E58 **Dietary calcium deficiency**

E58.XX   Oral manifestations

E60 **Dietary zinc deficiency**

E60.XX   Oral manifestations

E61 **Deficiency of other nutrient elements**

E61.VX   Oral manifestations

Obesity and other hyperalimentation

E67 **Other hyperalimentation**

E67.1   **Hypercarotenaemia**
E67.1X   Oral manifestations

E67.3   **Hypervitaminosis D**
E67.3X   Oral manifestations

Metabolic disorders

Excludes: Ehlers–Danlos syndrome (Q79.6)

E70 **Disorders of aromatic amino-acid metabolism**

E70.0   **Classical phenylketonuria**
E70.0X   Oral manifestations

E71 **Disorders of branched-chain amino-acid metabolism and fatty-acid metabolism**

E71.0   **Maple-syrup-urine disease**
E71.0X   Oral manifestations

E74 **Other disorders of carbohydrate metabolism**

E74.0   **Glycogen storage disease**
Includes: von Gierke's disease
E74.0X   Oral manifestations

E74.2   **Disorders of galactose metabolism**
Includes: galactosaemia
E74.2X   Oral manifestations

E74.9 **Disorder of carbohydrate metabolism, unspecified**
E74.9X Oral manifestations

E75 Disorders of sphingolipid metabolism and other lipid storage disorders

E75.2 **Other sphingolipidosis**
E75.20 Fabry(–Anderson) disease
E75.21 Gaucher's disease
E75.22 Niemann–Pick disease

E76 Disorders of glycosaminoglycan metabolism

Includes: Hurler's syndrome
Morquio's syndrome
E76.VX Oral manifestations

E78 Disorders of lipoprotein metabolism and other lipidaemias

E78.8 **Other disorders of lipoprotein metabolism**
Includes: Urbach–Wiethe disease
E78.8X Oral manifestations

E79 Disorders of purine and pyrimidine metabolism

E79.1 **Lesch–Nyhan syndrome**
E79.1X Oral manifestations

E80 Disorders of porphyrin and bilirubin metabolism

E80.0 **Hereditary erythropoietic porphyria**
E80.0X Oral manifestations

E80.3 **Defects of catalase and peroxidase**
E80.3X Oral manifestations of acatalasia

E83 Disorders of mineral metabolism

E83.1 **Disorders of iron metabolism**
Includes: haemochromatosis
E83.1X Oral manifestations

E83.2 **Disorders of zinc metabolism**
Includes: acrodermatitis enteropathica
E83.2X Oral manifestations

E83.3 **Disorders of phosphorus metabolism**
E83.30   Oral manifestations of hypophosphatasia
E83.31   Oral manifestations of vitamin-D-resistant rickets

E83.5 **Disorders of calcium metabolism**
Excludes: hyperparathyroidism (E21.0–E21.3)
E83.5X   Oral manifestations

E84 Cystic fibrosis

E84.VX   Oral manifestations

E85 Amyloidosis

E85.VX   Oral manifestations

CHAPTER V

Mental and behavioural disorders

Neurotic, stress-related and somatoform disorders

F45   Somatoform disorders

F45.8   **Other somatoform disorders**
        F45.80   Dysphagia, psychogenic
        F45.81   Torticollis, psychogenic
        F45.82   Teeth grinding [bruxism]

Behavioural syndromes associated with physiological disturbances and physical factors

F50   Eating disorders

     Includes: anorexia nervosa
                 bulimia
     F50.VX   Oral manifestations

Disorders of psychological development

F80   Specific developmental disorders of speech and language

F80.0   **Specific speech articulation disorder**
     Excludes: lisping (F80.8X)

F80.8   **Other developmental disorders of speech and language**
        F80.8X   Lisping

Behavioural and emotional disorders with onset usually occurring in childhood and adolescence

F98 Other behavioural and emotional disorders with onset usually occurring in childhood and adolescence

F98.5 Stuttering [stammering]

F98.8 Other specified behavioural and emotional disorders with onset usually occurring in childhood and adolescence
F98.8X   Thumb-sucking

CHAPTER VI

Diseases of the nervous system

Systemic atrophies primarily affecting the central nervous system

G12   Spinal muscular atrophy and related syndromes

G12.2   Motor neuron disease
Includes: amyotrophic lateral sclerosis
G12.2X   Oral manifestations

Extrapyramidal and movement disorders

G24   Dystonia

G24.3   Spasmodic torticollis

G24.4   Idiopathic orofacial dystonia

Episodic and paroxysmal disorders

G40   Epilepsy

G40.VX   Oral manifestations

G43   Migraine

G43.VX   Oral manifestations

Nerve, nerve root and plexus disorders

Excludes: neuralgia ⎫
            neuritis ⎬ NOS (M79.2)

G50 Disorders of trigeminal nerve

G50.0 **Trigeminal neuralgia**
Tic douloureux

G50.1 **Atypical facial pain**

G50.8 **Other disorders of trigeminal nerve**

G50.9 **Disorder of trigeminal nerve, unspecified**

G51 Facial nerve disorders

G51.0 **Bell's palsy**

G51.2 **Melkersson's syndrome**
Includes: Melkersson–Rosenthal syndrome
G51.2X   Oral manifestations

G51.3 **Clonic hemifacial spasm**

G51.4 **Facial myokymia**

G51.8 **Other specified facial nerve disorders**

G51.9 **Disorder of facial nerve, unspecified**

G52 Disorders of other cranial nerves

G52.1 **Disorders of glossopharyngeal nerve**
G52.1X   Glossopharyngeal neuralgia

G52.3 **Disorders of hypoglossal nerve**
12th cranial nerve

G52.9 **Cranial nerve disorder, unspecified**

Other disorders of the nervous system

G90 Disorders of autonomic nervous system

G90.1 **Familial dysautonomia [Riley–Day]**
G90.1X   Oral manifestations

G90.2 **Horner's syndrome**
G90.2X   Oral manifestations

CHAPTER IX

Diseases of the circulatory system

Diseases of arteries, arterioles and capillaries

I78   Diseases of capillaries

I78.0   **Hereditary haemorrhagic telangiectasia**
Includes: Rendu–Osler–Weber disease
I78.0X   Oral manifestations

Diseases of veins, lymphatic vessels and lymph nodes, not elsewhere classified

I86   Varicose veins of other sites

I86.0   **Sublingual varices**

I87   Other disorders of veins

I87.8   **Other specified disorders of veins**
Includes: phlebolith
I87.8X   Oral manifestations

I88   Nonspecific lymphadenitis

I88.1   **Chronic lymphadenitis, except mesenteric**
I88.1X   Head and neck

CHAPTER X

Diseases of the respiratory system

Acute upper respiratory infections

J01 **Acute sinusitis**

J01.0   **Acute maxillary sinusitis**

J01.1   **Acute frontal sinusitis**

J01.9   **Acute sinusitis, unspecified**

J03 **Acute tonsillitis**

Influenza and pneumonia

J10 **Influenza due to identified influenza virus**

J10.1   **Influenza with other respiratory manifestations, influenza virus identified**
       J10.1X   Oral manifestations

J11 **Influenza, virus not identified**

J11.1   **Influenza with other respiratory manifestations, virus not identified**
       J11.1X   Oral manifestations

Other diseases of upper respiratory tract

J32 **Chronic sinusitis**

J32.0   **Chronic maxillary sinusitis**

J32.1   **Chronic frontal sinusitis**

J32.9   **Chronic sinusitis, unspecified**

J33 Nasal polyp

J33.8 **Other polyp of sinus**
J33.8X   Polyp of maxillary sinus

J34 Other disorders of nose and nasal sinuses

J34.1 **Cyst and mucocele of nasal sinus**
J34.1X   Cyst and mucocele of maxillary sinus

J35 Chronic diseases of tonsils and adenoids

J35.0 **Chronic tonsillitis**

J36 Peritonsillar abscess

CHAPTER XI

Diseases of the digestive system

Diseases of oral cavity, salivary glands and jaws

K00   Disorders of tooth development and eruption

Excludes: embedded and impacted teeth (K01.–)

K00.0   Anodontia
K00.00   Partial anodontia [hypodontia] [oligodontia]
K00.01   Total anodontia
K00.09   Anodontia, unspecified

K00.1   Supernumerary teeth
Includes: supplementary teeth
Excludes: impacted supernumerary teeth (K01.18)
K00.10   Incisor and canine regions
   Mesiodens
K00.11   Premolar region
K00.12   Molar region
   Distomolar
   Fourth molar
   Paramolar
K00.19   Supernumerary teeth, unspecified

K00.2   Abnormalities of size and form of teeth
K00.20   Macrodontia
K00.21   Microdontia
K00.22   Concrescence
K00.23   Fusion and gemination
   Schizodontia
   Synodontia
K00.24   Dens evaginatus [occlusal tuberculum]
   Excludes: tuberculum Carabelli, which is regarded as a
      normal variation and should not be coded
K00.25   Dens invaginatus ["dens in dente"] [dilated
   odontoma] and incisor anomalies
   Palatal groove
   Peg-shaped [conical] incisors
   Shovel-shaped incisors
   T-shaped incisors

K00.26 Premolarization

K00.27 Abnormal tubercula and enamel pearls [enameloma]

Excludes: dens evaginatus [occlusal tuberculum] (K00.24)
tuberculum Carabelli, which is regarded as a
normal variation and should not be coded

K00.28 Taurodontism

K00.29 Other and unspecified abnormalities of size and form of teeth

K00.3 Mottled teeth

Excludes: deposits [accretions] on teeth (K03.6)
Turner's tooth (K00.46)

K00.30 Endemic (fluoride) mottling of enamel [dental fluorosis]

K00.31 Non-endemic mottling of enamel [non-fluoride enamel opacities]

K00.39 Mottled teeth, unspecified

K00.4 Disturbances in tooth formation

Excludes: hereditary disturbances in tooth structure (K00.5)
Hutchinson's incisors (A50.51)
mottled teeth (K00.3)
mulberry molars (A50.52)

K00.40 Enamel hypoplasia

K00.41 Prenatal enamel hypoplasia

K00.42 Neonatal enamel hypoplasia

K00.43 Aplasia and hypoplasia of cementum

K00.44 Dilaceration

K00.45 Odontodysplasia [regional odontodysplasia]

K00.46 Turner's tooth

K00.48 Other specified disturbances in tooth formation

K00.49 Disturbance in tooth formation, unspecified

K00.5 Hereditary disturbances in tooth structure, not elsewhere classified

K00.50 Amelogenesis imperfecta

K00.51 Dentinogenesis imperfecta

Dental changes in osteogenesis imperfecta (78.0)

Excludes: dentinal dysplasia (K00.58)
shell teeth (K00.58)

K00.52 Odontogenesis imperfecta

K00.58   Other hereditary disturbances in tooth structure
Dentinal dysplasia
Shell teeth
K00.59   Hereditary disturbances in tooth structure,
unspecified

K00.6   Disturbances in tooth eruption
K00.60   Natal teeth
K00.61   Neonatal teeth
K00.62   Premature eruption [dentia praecox]
K00.63   Retained [persistent] primary [deciduous] teeth
K00.64   Late eruption
K00.65   Premature shedding of primary [deciduous] teeth
Excludes: exfoliation of teeth (attributable to disease
of surrounding tissues) (K08.0X)
K00.68   Other specified disturbances in tooth eruption
K00.69   Disturbance in tooth eruption, unspecified

K00.7   Teething syndrome

K00.8   Other disorders of tooth development
Includes: intrinsic staining of teeth NOS
Excludes: discolorations of local origin (K03.6, K03.7)
K00.80   Colour changes during tooth formation due to
blood type incompatibility
K00.81   Colour changes during tooth formation due to
malformation of biliary system
K00.82   Colour changes during tooth formation due to
porphyria
K00.83   Colour changes during tooth formation due to
tetracyclines
K00.88   Other specified disorders of tooth development

K00.9   Disorders of tooth development, unspecified

K01   Embedded and impacted teeth

Excludes: embedded and impacted teeth with abnormal position of
such teeth or adjacent teeth (K07.3)

K01.0   Embedded teeth
An embedded tooth is a tooth that has failed to erupt without
obstruction by another tooth.

K01.1   Impacted teeth
An impacted tooth is a tooth that has failed to erupt because of
obstruction by another tooth.
K01.10   Maxillary incisor

K01.11 Mandibular incisor
K01.12 Maxillary canine
K01.13 Mandibular canine
K01.14 Maxillary premolar
K01.15 Mandibular premolar
K01.16 Maxillary molar
K01.17 Mandibular molar
K01.18 Supernumerary tooth
K01.19 Impacted tooth, unspecified

K02 Dental caries

K02.0 Caries limited to enamel
White spot lesion [initial caries]

K02.1 Caries extending into dentine

K02.2 Caries of cementum

K02.3 Arrested caries

K02.4 Odontoclasia
Infantile melanodontia
Melanodontoclasia
Excludes: internal and external resorption of teeth (K03.3)

K02.8 Other specified dental caries

K02.9 Dental caries, unspecified

K03 Other diseases of hard tissues of teeth

Excludes: bruxism (F45.8)
dental caries (K02.–)
teeth-grinding (F45.8)

K03.0 Excessive attrition of teeth
K03.00 Occlusal
K03.01 Approximal
K03.08 Other specified attrition of teeth
K03.09 Attrition of teeth, unspecified

K03.1 Abrasion of teeth
K03.10 Dentifrice
Wedge defect NOS
K03.11 Habitual
K03.12 Occupational
K03.13 Traditional
Ritual

K03.18   Other specified abrasion of teeth

K03.19   Abrasion of teeth, unspecified

K03.2   Erosion of teeth

K03.20   Occupational

K03.21   Due to persistent regurgitating or vomiting

K03.22   Due to diet

K03.23   Due to drugs and medicaments

K03.24   Idiopathic

K03.28   Other specified erosion of teeth

K03.29   Erosion of teeth, unspecified

K03.3   Pathological resorption of teeth

K03.30   External

K03.31   Internal [internal granuloma] [pink spot]

K03.39   Pathological resorption of teeth, unspecified

K03.4   Hypercementosis

Excludes: hypercementosis in Paget's disease

K03.5   Ankylosis of teeth

K03.6   Deposits [accretions] on teeth

Includes: staining of teeth NOS

K03.60   Pigmented film

Black

Green

Orange

K03.61   Due to tobacco habit

K03.62   Due to betel-chewing habit

K03.63   Other gross soft deposits

Materia alba

K03.64   Supragingival calculus

K03.65   Subgingival calculus

K03.66   Dental plaque

K03.68   Other specified deposits on teeth

K03.69   Deposit on teeth, unspecified

K03.7   Posteruptive colour changes of dental hard tissues

Excludes: deposits [accretions] on teeth (K03.6)

K03.70   Due to metals and metallic compounds

K03.71   Due to pulpal bleeding

K03.72   Due to chewing habit

Betel

Tobacco

K03.78   Other specified colour changes

K03.79   Colour change, unspecified

K03.8 **Other specified diseases of hard tissues of teeth**
  K03.80 Sensitive dentine
  K03.81 Changes in enamel due to irradiation
      Use additional external cause code (Chapter XX), if desired,
      to identify radiation.
  K03.88 Other specified diseases of hard tissues of teeth

K03.9 **Disease of hard tissues of teeth, unspecified**

K04 Diseases of pulp and periapical tissues

K04.0 **Pulpitis**
  K04.00 Initial (hyperaemia)
  K04.01 Acute
  K04.02 Suppurative [pulpal abscess]
  K04.03 Chronic
  K04.04 Chronic, ulcerative
  K04.05 Chronic, hyperplastic [pulpal polyp]
  K04.08 Other specified pulpitis
  K04.09 Pulpitis, unspecified

K04.1 **Necrosis of pulp**
  Pulpal gangrene

K04.2 **Pulp degeneration**
  Denticles
  Pulpal calcification
  Pulpal stones

K04.3 **Abnormal hard tissue formation in pulp**
  K04.3X Secondary or irregular dentine
      Excludes: pulpal calcifications (K04.2)
          pulpal stones (K04.2)

K04.4 **Acute apical periodontitis of pulpal origin**
  Acute apical periodontitis NOS

K04.5 **Chronic apical periodontitis**
  Apical granuloma

K04.6 **Periapical abscess with sinus**
  Includes: dental
      dentoalveolar } abscess with sinus
      periodontal abscess of pulpal origin
  K04.60 Sinus to maxillary antrum
  K04.61 Sinus to nasal cavity
  K04.62 Sinus to oral cavity

K04.63 Sinus to skin
K04.69 Periapical abscess with sinus, unspecified

K04.7 Periapical abscess without sinus
Dental abscess
Dentoalveolar abscess   } without sinus
Periodontal abscess of pulpal origin
Periapical abscess with no reference to sinus

K04.8 Radicular cyst
Includes: cyst
   • apical periodontal
   • periapical
K04.80 Apical and lateral
K04.81 Residual
K04.82 Inflammatory paradental
        Excludes: developmental lateral periodontal cyst (K09.04)
K04.89 Radicular cyst, unspecified

K04.9 Other and unspecified diseases of pulp and periapical tissues

K05 Gingivitis and periodontal diseases

Includes: disease of edentulous alveolar ridge

K05.0 Acute gingivitis
Excludes: acute pericoronitis (K05.22)
        acute necrotizing ulcerative gingivitis [fusospirochaetal gingivitis] [Vincent's gingivitis] (A69.10)
        herpesviral gingivostomatitis (B00.2X)
K05.00 Acute streptococcal gingivostomatitis
K05.08 Other specified acute gingivitis
K05.09 Acute gingivitis, unspecified

K05.1 Chronic gingivitis
K05.10 Simple marginal
K05.11 Hyperplastic
K05.12 Ulcerative
        Excludes: necrotizing ulcerative gingivitis (A69.10)
K05.13 Desquamative
K05.18 Other specified chronic gingivitis
K05.19 Chronic gingivitis, unspecified

K05.2 Acute periodontitis

    K05.20 Periodontal abscess [parodontal abscess] of gingival origin without sinus

      Periodontal abscess of gingival origin with no reference to sinus

      Excludes: acute apical periodontitis of pulpal origin (K04.4)

         acute periapical abscess of pulpal origin (K04.6, K04.7)

    K05.21 Periodontal abscess [parodontal abscess] of gingival origin with sinus

      Excludes: acute apical periodontitis of pulpal origin (K04.4)

         acute periapical abscess of pulpal origin (K04.6, K04.7)

    K05.22 Acute pericoronitis

    K05.28 Other specified acute periodontitis

    K05.29 Acute periodontitis, unspecified

K05.3 Chronic periodontitis

    K05.30 Simplex

    K05.31 Complex

    K05.32 Chronic pericoronitis

    K05.33 Thickened follicle

    K05.38 Other specified chronic periodontitis

    K05.39 Chronic periodontitis, unspecified

K05.4 Periodontosis

Juvenile periodontosis

K05.5 Other periodontal diseases

K06 Other disorders of gingiva and edentulous alveolar ridge

Excludes: atrophy of edentulous alveolar ridge (K08.2)

      gingivitis (K05.0, K05.1)

K06.0 Gingival recession

Includes: postinfective

       postoperative

    K06.00 Localized

    K06.01 Generalized

    K06.09 Gingival recession, unspecified

K06.1 **Gingival enlargement**
Includes: tuberosity
K06.10 Gingival fibromatosis
K06.18 Other specified gingival enlargement
K06.19 Gingival enlargement, unspecified

K06.2 **Gingival and edentulous alveolar ridge lesions associated with trauma**
K06.20 Due to traumatic occlusion
K06.21 Due to toothbrushing
K06.22 Frictional [functional] keratosis
K06.23 Irritative hyperplasia [denture hyperplasia]
K06.28 Other specified gingival and edentulous alveolar ridge lesions associated with trauma
K06.29 Unspecified gingival and edentulous alveolar ridge lesions associated with trauma

K06.8 **Other specified disorders of gingiva and edentulous alveolar ridge**
K06.80 Gingival cyst of adult
Excludes: gingival cyst of newborn (K09.82)
K06.81 Peripheral giant cell granuloma [giant cell epulis]
K06.82 Fibrous epulis
K06.83 Pyogenic granuloma
Excludes: pyogenic granuloma of site other than gingiva or edentulous alveolar ridge (K13.40)
K06.84 Flabby ridge
K06.88 Other

K06.9 **Disorder of gingiva and edentulous alveolar ridge, unspecified**

K07 Dentofacial anomalies [including malocclusion]

K07.0 **Major anomalies of jaw size**
Excludes: acromegaly (E22.0)
hemifacial atrophy or hypertrophy (Q67.4)
Robin's syndrome (Q87.0)
unilateral condylar hyperplasia (K10.81)
unilateral condylar hypoplasia (K10.82)
K07.00 Maxillary macrognathism [maxillary hyperplasia]
K07.01 Mandibular macrognathism [mandibular hyperplasia]
K07.02 Macrognathism, both jaws
K07.03 Maxillary micrognathism [maxillary hypoplasia]
K07.04 Mandibular micrognathism [mandibular hypoplasia]

K07.05   Micrognathism, both jaws
K07.08   Other specified jaw size anomalies
K07.09   Anomaly of jaw size, unspecified

K07.1   Anomalies of jaw–cranial base relationship
K07.10   Asymmetries
Excludes: hemifacial atrophy (Q64.40)
hemifacial hypertrophy (Q67.41)
unilateral condylar hyperplasia (K10.81)
unilateral condylar hypoplasia (K10.82)
K07.11   Mandibular prognathism
K07.12   Maxillary prognathism
K07.13   Mandibular retrognathism
K07.14   Maxillary retrognathism
K07.18   Other specified anomalies of jaw–cranial base relationship
K07.19   Anomaly of jaw–cranial base relationship, unspecified

K07.2   Anomalies of dental arch relationship
K07.20   Disto-occlusion
K07.21   Mesio-occlusion
K07.22   Excessive overjet [horizontal overbite]
K07.23   Excessive overbite [vertical overbite]
K07.24   Openbite
K07.25   Crossbite (anterior, posterior)
K07.26   Midline deviation
K07.27   Posterior lingual occlusion of mandibular teeth
K07.28   Other specified anomalies of dental arch relation-ship
K07.29   Anomaly of dental arch relationship, unspecified

K07.3   Anomalies of tooth position
K07.30   Crowding
Imbrication
K07.31   Displacement
K07.32   Rotation
K07.33   Spacing
Diastema
K07.34   Transposition
K07.35   Embedded or impacted teeth in abnormal position
Excludes: embedded or impacted teeth in normal position (K01.0, K01.1)
K07.38   Other specified anomalies of tooth position
K07.39   Anomaly of tooth position, unspecified

K07.4   Malocclusion, unspecified

K07.5   Dentofacial functional abnormalities
Excludes: bruxism [teeth-grinding] (F45.82)
K07.50   Abnormal jaw closure
K07.51   Malocclusion due to abnormal swallowing
K07.54   Malocclusion due to mouth breathing
K07.55   Malocclusion due to tongue, lip or finger habits
K07.58   Other specified dentofacial functional abnormalities
K07.59   Dentofacial functional abnormality, unspecified

K07.6   Temporomandibular joint disorders
K07.60   Temporomandibular joint-pain-dysfunction
          syndrome [Costen]
          Excludes: current temporomandibular joint dislocation
              (S03.0) and strain (S03.4)
              diseases listed in Chapter XIII
K07.61   Clicking (snapping) jaws
K07.62   Recurrent dislocation and subluxation of temporo-
          mandibular joint
          Excludes: current injury (S03.0)
K07.63   Pain in temporomandibular joint, not elsewhere
          classified
          Excludes: temporomandibular joint-pain-dysfunction
              syndrome [Costen] (K07.60)
K07.64   Stiffness of temporomandibular joint, not elsewhere
          classified
K07.65   Osteophyte of temporomandibular joint
K07.68   Other specified temporomandibular joint disorders
K07.69   Temporomandibular joint disorder, unspecified

K08   Other disorders of teeth and supporting structures

K08.0   Exfoliation of teeth due to systemic causes
Excludes: anodontia (K00.0)
K08.0X   Exfoliation of teeth (attributable to disease of
          surrounding tissues, including systemic causes,
          e.g. acrodynia (T56.1), hypophosphatasia (E83.3))
          Excludes: premature shedding of primary [deciduous]
              teeth (K00.65)

**K08.1   Loss of teeth due to accident, extraction or local periodontal
          disease**
Excludes: Current accident (S03.2)

K08.2   Atrophy of edentulous alveolar ridge

K08.3   **Retained dental root**

K08.8   **Other specified disorders of teeth and supporting structures**
K08.80   Toothache NOS
K08.81   Irregular alveolar process
K08.82   Enlargement of alveolar ridge NOS
K08.88   Other

K08.9   **Disorder of teeth and supporting structures, unspecified**

K09   Cysts of oral region, not elsewhere classified

Excludes: radicular cyst (K04.8)
           mucous cyst (K11.6)

K09.0   **Developmental odontogenic cysts[1]**
K09.00   Eruption
K09.01   Gingival
K09.02   Keratocyst [primordial]
K09.03   Follicular [dentigerous]
K09.04   Lateral periodontal
K09.08   Other specified developmental odontogenic cysts
K09.09   Developmental odontogenic cyst, unspecified

K09.1   **Developmental (nonodontogenic) cysts of oral region[1]**
Includes: "fissural" cysts
K09.10   Globulomaxillary
K09.11   Median palatal
K09.12   Nasopalatine [incisive canal]
K09.13   Palatine papilla
K09.18   Other specified developmental cysts of oral region
K09.19   Developmental cyst of oral region, unspecified

K09.2   **Other cysts of jaw[1]**
Excludes: latent bone cyst of jaw (K10.02)
           Stafne's cyst (K10.02)
K09.20   Aneurysmal bone cyst[2]
K09.21   Solitary bone [traumatic] [haemorrhagic] cyst
K09.22   Epithelial jaw cysts not identifiable as odontogenic or nonodontogenic
K09.28   Other specified cysts of jaw
K09.29   Cyst of jaw, unspecified

---

[1] See pages 5 and 132–143 and Annex 1, page 144.
[2] Lesions showing histological features both of aneurysmal cyst and of another fibro-osseous lesion should be classified here.

K09.8 Other cysts of oral region, not elsewhere classified
K09.80 Dermoid cyst
K09.81 Epidermoid cyst
K09.82 Gingival cyst of newborn
Excludes: gingival cyst of adult (K06.80)
K09.83 Palatal cyst of newborn
Epstein's pearl
K09.84 Nasoalveolar [nasolabial] cyst
K09.85 Lymphoepithelial cyst
K09.88 Other specified cysts of oral region

K09.9 Cyst of oral region, unspecified

K10 Other diseases of jaws

K10.0 Developmental disorders of jaws
K10.00 Torus mandibularis
K10.01 Torus palatinus
K10.02 Latent bone cyst
Developmental bone defect in mandible
Stafne's cyst
Static bone cyst
K10.08 Other specified developmental disorders of jaws
K10.09 Developmental disorder of jaws, unspecified

K10.1 Giant cell granuloma, central
Giant cell granuloma NOS
Excludes: peripheral (K06.81)

K10.2 Inflammatory conditions of jaws
Use additional external cause code (Chapter XX), if desired, to identify radiation, if radiation-induced.
K10.20 Osteitis of jaw
Excludes: alveolar osteitis (K10.3)
dry socket (K10.3)
K10.21 Osteomyelitis of jaw
Excludes: neonatal osteomyelitis of maxilla [neonatal maxillitis] (K10.24)
K10.22 Periostitis of jaw
K10.23 Chronic periostitis of jaw
Hyaline microangiopathy
Pulse granuloma
K10.24 Neonatal osteomyelitis of maxilla [neonatal maxillitis]
K10.25 Sequestrum
K10.26 Osteoradionecrosis

K10.28 Other specified inflammatory conditions of jaws
K10.29 Inflammatory condition of jaws, unspecified

K10.3 Alveolitis of jaws
Alveolar osteitis
Dry socket

K10.8 Other specified diseases of jaws
Excludes: fibrous dysplasia, polyostotic (Q78.1)
K10.80 Cherubism[1]
K10.81 Unilateral condylar hyperplasia of mandible
K10.82 Unilateral condylar hypoplasia of mandible
K10.83 Fibrous dysplasia of jaw
K10.88 Other specified diseases of jaws
Exostosis of jaw

K10.9 Disease of jaws, unspecified

K11   Diseases of salivary glands

Excludes: salivary gland tumours (C07.–, C08.–, D10.–, D11.–)

K11.0 Atrophy of salivary gland

K11.1 Hypertrophy of salivary gland

K11.2 Sialoadenitis
Excludes: epidemic parotitis [mumps] (B26.–)
        uveoparotid fever [Heerfordt] (D86.8)

K11.3 Abscess of salivary gland

K11.4 Fistula of salivary gland
Excludes: congenital fistula of salivary gland (Q38.43)

K11.5 Sialolithiasis
Calculus [stone] in salivary duct

K11.6 Mucocele of salivary gland
Ranula
K11.60 Mucous retention cyst
K11.61 Mucous extravasation cyst
K11.69 Mucocele of salivary gland, unspecified

K11.7 Disturbances of salivary secretion
Excludes: dry mouth NOS (R68.2)
        sicca syndrome [Sjögren] (M35.0)
K11.70 Hyposecretion

---

[1]See pages 5 and 132–143 and Annex 2, page 147.

K11.71 Xerostomia
K11.72 Hypersecretion [ptyalism]
K11.78 Other specified disturbances of salivary secretion
K11.79 Disturbance of salivary secretion, unspecified

K11.8 Other diseases of salivary glands
Excludes: sicca syndrome [Sjögren] (M35.0)
K11.80 Benign lymphoepithelial lesion of salivary gland
K11.81 Mikulicz' disease
K11.82 Stenosis [stricture] of salivary duct
K11.83 Sialectasia
K11.84 Sialosis
K11.85 Necrotizing sialometaplasia
K11.88 Other specified diseases of salivary glands

K11.9 Disease of salivary gland, unspecified
Sialoadenopathy NOS

K12 Stomatitis and related lesions

Excludes: focal epithelial hyperplasia (B07.X2)
herpangina (B08.5X)
pyostomatitis vegetans (L08.0X) stomatitis:
• acute necrotizing (A69.0)
• allergic (L23.–)
• candidal (B37.0)
• cotton roll (K12.14)
• Coxsackievirus NOS (B34.1)
• epizootic (B08.8)
• fusospirochaetal (A69.0)
• medicamentosa (T36–T50)
• mycotic (B37.0)
• nicotinic (K13.24)
• vesicular with exanthem (B08.4)
streptococcal gingivostomatitis (K05.00)
vesicular stomatitis virus disease [Indiana fever]
  (A93.8X)

K12.0 Recurrent oral aphthae
K12.00 Recurrent (minor) aphthae
        Aphthous stomatitis
        Canker sore
        Mikulicz' aphthae
        Minor aphthae
        Recurrent aphthous ulcer

K12.01 Periadenitis mucosa necrotica recurrens
Cicatrizing aphthous stomatitis
Major aphthae
Sutton's aphthae

K12.02 Stomatitis herpetiformis [herpetiform eruption]
Excludes: dermatitis herpetiformis (L13.0X)
herpesviral gingivostomatitis (B00.2X)

K12.03 Bednar's aphthae

K12.04 Traumatic ulcer
Excludes: traumatic ulcer of tongue (K14.01)
ulcers of tongue NOS (K14.09)

K12.08 Other specified recurrent oral aphthae

K12.09 Recurrent oral aphthae, unspecified

K12.1 Other forms of stomatitis

K12.10 Stomatitis artifacta

K12.11 Geographic stomatitis
Excludes: geographic tongue (K14.1)

K12.12 Denture stomatitis
Excludes: denture stomatitis due to candidal infection (B37.03)
traumatic ulcer due to denture (K12.04)

K12.13 Papillary hyperplasia of palate

K12.14 Contact stomatitis
Cotton roll stomatitis

K12.18 Other specified forms of stomatitis

K12.19 Stomatitis, unspecified

K12.2 Cellulitis and abscess of mouth
Phlegmon
Submandibular abscess
Excludes: abscess (of):
• periapical (K04.6–K04.7)
• periodontal (K05.21)
• peritonsillar (J36)
• salivary gland (K11.3)
• tongue (K14.00)

K13 Other diseases of lip and oral mucosa

Includes: epithelial disturbances of tongue
Excludes: certain disorders of gingiva and edentulous alveolar ridge (K05–K06)
cysts of oral region (K09.–)
diseases of tongue (K14.–)
stomatitis and related lesions (K12.–)

K13.0   Diseases of lips
Excludes: actinic cheilitis (L56.8X)
a ariboflavinosis (E53.0)

    K13.00   Angular cheilitis
        Angular cheilosis
        Perlèche NEC
        Excludes: perlèche due to:
            • candidiasis (B37.0)
            • riboflavin deficiency (E53.0)

    K13.01   Cheilitis glandularis apostematosa
    K13.02   Cheilitis, exfoliative
    K13.03   Cheilitis NOS
    K13.04   Cheilodynia
    K13.08   Other specified diseases of lips
    K13.09   Disease of lips, unspecified

K13.1   Cheek and lip biting

K13.2[1]   Leukoplakia and other disturbances of oral epithelium, including tongue
Excludes: candidal leukoplakia (B37.02)
aa focal epithelial hyperplasia (B07.X2)
aa frictional keratosis (K06.22)
aa functional keratosis (K06.22)
aa hairy leukoplakia (K13.3)

    K13.20   Leukoplakia, idiopathic
    K13.21   Leukoplakia, tobacco-associated
        Excludes: leukokeratosis nicotina palati (K13.24)
            smoker's palate (K13.24)

    K13.22   Erythroplakia
    K13.23   Leukoedema

---

[1]Lesions (such as leukoplakia, erythroplakia) without reference to severe dysplasia are assigned to this section, and the following 6th character coding may be used

0 Stated to be without dysplasia (or Grade 0)

1 Slight (mild) dysplasia (or Grade 1)

2 Moderate dysplasia (or Grade 2)

9 No reference to dysplasia

Lesions with mention of severe dysplasia (or Grades 3 or 4) are assigned to the section on in-situ neoplasms (D00–D09).

For the purposes of this classification, leukoplakia is defined as a white lesion of the oral mucosa that cannot be placed in any other listed diagnostic category.

K13.24   Smoker's palate [leukokeratosis nicotina palati]
[nicotinic stomatitis]
K13.28   Other
K13.29   Unspecified
Leukoplakia NOS

K13.3   Hairy leukoplakia

K13.4   Granuloma and granuloma-like lesions of oral mucosa
K13.40   Pyogenic granuloma
Excludes: gingiva (K06.83)
K13.41   Eosinophilic granuloma of oral mucosa
Excludes: eosinophilic granuloma of bone (D76.00)
histiocytosis X (D76. –)
K13.42   Verrucous xanthoma [histiocytosis Y]
K13.48   Other specified granuloma and granuloma-like
lesions of oral mucosa
K13.49   Granuloma and granuloma-like lesions of oral
mucosa, unspecified

K13.5   Oral submucous fibrosis

K13.6   Irritative hyperplasia of oral mucosa
Excludes: irritative hyperplasia [denture hyperplasia] of
edentulous alveolar ridge (K06.23)

K13.7   Other and unspecified lesions of oral mucosa
K13.70   Excessive melanin pigmentation
Melanoplakia
Smoker's melanosis
K13.71   Oral fistula
Excludes: oroantral fistula (T81.8)
K13.72   Deliberate tattoo
Excludes: amalgam tattoo (T81.50)
K13.73   Focal oral mucinosis
K13.78   Other specified lesions of oral mucosa
Linea alba
K13.79   Lesion of oral mucosa, unspecified

K14   Diseases of tongue

Excludes: erythroplakia of tongue (K13.22)
focal epithelial hyperplasia (B07.X2)
hairy leukoplakia (K13.3)
leukoedema ⎱
leukoplakia ⎰ of tongue (K13.2)
macroglossia (congenital) (Q38.2X)
submucous fibrosis of tongue (K13.5)

K14.0 Glossitis
Excludes: atrophic glossitis (K14.42)
K14.00   Abscess of tongue
K14.01   Traumatic ulceration of tongue
K14.08   Other specified glossitis
K14.09   Glossitis, unspecified
        Ulcer of tongue NOS

K14.1 Geographic tongue
Benign migratory glossitis
Glossitis areata exfoliativa

K14.2 Median rhomboid glossitis

K14.3 Hypertrophy of tongue papillae
K14.30   Coated tongue
K14.31   Hairy tongue
        Black hairy tongue
        Lingua villosa nigra
        Excludes: hairy leukoplakia (K13.3)
                    hairy tongue due to antibiotics (K14.38)
K14.32   Hypertrophy of foliate papillae
K14.38   Other specified hypertrophy of tongue papillae
        Hairy tongue due to antibiotics
K14.39   Hypertrophy of tongue papillae, unspecified

K14.5 Plicated tongue
Fissured
Furrowed   } tongue
Scrotal
Excludes: fissured tongue, congenital (Q38.33)

K14.6 Glossodynia
Excludes: abnormalities of taste (R43.–)
K14.60   Glossopyrosis [burning tongue]
K14.61   Glossodynia [painful tongue]
K14.68   Other specified glossodynia
K16.49   Glossodynia, unspecfied

K14.8 Other diseases of tongue
K14.80   Crenated tongue [lingua indentata]
K14.81   Hypertrophy of tongue
        Hemihypertrophy of tongue
        Excludes: macroglossia (congenital) (Q38.2X)
K14.82   Atrophy of tongue
        Hemiatrophy of tongue
        Excludes: atrophy of tongue papillae (K14.4)

K14.88　Other specified diseases of tongue
Diseases of lingual tonsil

K14.9　Disease of tongue, unspecified

Noninfective enteritis and colitis

K50　Crohn's disease [regional enteritis]

K50.8X　Oral manifestations

CHAPTER XII

Diseases of the skin and subcutaneous tissue

Infections of the skin and subcutaneous tissue

L02 Cutaneous abscess, furuncle and carbuncle

L02.0 Cutaneous abscess, furuncle and carbuncle of face

L02.1 Cutaneous abscess, furuncle and carbuncle of neck

L03 Cellulitis

Excludes: cellulitis of mouth (K12.2X)

L03.2 Cellulitis of face

L03.8 Cellulitis of other sites
L03.8X   Head and neck [any part, except face]

L04 Acute lymphadenitis

Includes: abscess (acute) of lymph node
Excludes: chronic lymphadenitis (I88.1)
enlarged lymph nodes NOS (R59. –)
HIV disease with generalized lymphadenopathy (B23.1)

L04.0 Acute lymphadenitis of face, head and neck

L08 Other local infections of skin and subcutaneous tissue

L08.0 Pyoderma
L08.0X   Pyostomatitis vegetans

L08.8 Other specified local infections of skin and subcutaneous tissue
L08.8X   Face and neck

Bullous disorders

Excludes: benign familial pemphigus [Hailey–Hailey] (Q82.80)

L10 Pemphigus

L10.0 **Pemphigus vulgaris**
L10.0X   Oral manifestations

L10.1 **Pemphigus vegetans**
L10.1X   Oral manifestations

L10.2 **Pemphigus foliaceus**
L10.2X   Oral manifestations

L10.5 **Drug-induced pemphigus**
L10.5X   Oral manifestations

L10.8 **Other pemphigus**
L10.8X   Oral manifestations

L10.9 **Pemphigus, unspecified**
L10.9X   Oral manifestations

L12 Pemphigoid

L12.0 **Bullous pemphigoid**
L12.0X   Oral manifestations

L12.1 **Cicatricial pemphigoid**
Includes: benign mucous membrane pemphigoid
L12.1X   Oral manifestations

L12.2 **Chronic bullous disease of childhood**
L12.2X   Oral manifestations

L12.3 **Acquired epidermolysis bullosa**
L12.3X   Oral manifestations

L12.8 **Other pemphigoid**
L12.8X   Oral manifestations

L12.9 **Pemphigoid, unspecified**
L12.9X   Oral manifestations

L13 Other bullous disorders

L13.0 **Dermatitis herpetiformis**
Includes: Dühring's disease
Excludes: stomatitis herpetiformis (K12.02)
L13.0X   Oral manifestations

L13.8   **Other specified bullous disorders**
          L13.8X   Oral manifestations

L13.9   **Bullous disorder, unspecified**
          L13.9X   Oral manifestations

Dermatitis and eczema

L23   Other allergic contact dermatitis

L23.2   **Allergic contact dermatitis due to cosmetics**
          L23.2X   Oral manifestations

L24   Irritant contact dermatitis

          Excludes: contact stomatitis (K12.14)
          L24.VX   Oral manifestations

Papulosquamous disorders

L40   Psoriasis

L40.0   **Psoriasis vulgaris**
          L40.0X   Oral manifestations

L40.1   **Generalized pustular psoriasis**
          L40.1X   Oral manifestations

L40.2   **Acrodermatitis continua**
          L40.2X   Oral manifestations

L42   Pityriasis rosea

          L42.XX   Oral manifestations

L43   Lichen planus

L43.1   **Bullous lichen planus**
          L43.1X   Oral manifestations

L43.2   **Lichenoid drug reaction**
          Use additional cause code (Chapter XX), if desired, to identify drug.
          L43.2X   Oral manifestations

L43.8   **Other lichen planus**
          L43.80   Oral manifestations of lichen planus, papular

L43.81   Oral manifestations of lichen planus, reticular
L43.82   Oral manifestations of lichen planus, atrophic and erosive
L43.83   Oral manifestations of lichen planus, plaque type
L43.88   Oral manifestations of other specified lichen planus
L43.89   Oral manifestation of unspecified lichen planus

Urticaria and erythema

L51 Erythema multiforme

L51.0   **Nonbullous erythema multiforme**
L51.0X   Oral manifestations

L51.1   **Bullous erythema multiforme**
Includes: Stevens–Johnson syndrome
L51.1X   Oral manifestations

L51.9   **Erythema multiforme, unspecified**
L51.9X   Oral manifestations

Radiation-related disorders of the skin and subcutaneous tissue

L56 Other acute skin changes due to ultraviolet radiation

L56.8   **Other specified acute skin changes due to ultraviolet radiation**
L56.8X   Actinic cheilitis

Disorders of skin appendages

L71 Rosacea

L71.0   **Perioral dermatitis**
Use additional external cause code (Chapter XX), if desired, to identify drug, if drug-induced.

Other disorders of the skin and subcutaneous tissue

L80 Vitiligo

L80.XX   Face and neck

L81 Other disorders of pigmentation

Excludes: naevi — see Alphabetical index
Peutz–Jeghers syndrome (Q85.80)

L81.3 Café au lait spots
L81.3X   Face and neck

L81.4 Other melanin hyperpigmentation
Includes: lentigo
L81.4X   Face and neck

L81.5 Leukoderma, not elsewhere classified
L81.5X   Face and neck

L81.8 Other specified disorders of pigmentation
L81.8X   Face and neck

L82 Seborrhoeic keratosis

L82.XX   Face and neck

L83 Ancanthosis nigricans

L83.XX   Face and neck

L85 Other epidermal thickening

L85.8 Other specified epidermal thickening
L85.8X   Keratoacanthoma

L90 Atrophic disorders of skin

L90.0 Lichen sclerosus et atrophicus
L90.0X   Oral manifestations

L91 Hypertrophic disorders of skin

L91.0 Keloid scar
L91.0X   Face and neck

L92 Granulomatous disorders of skin and subcutaneous tissue

L92.0 Granuloma annulare
L92.0X   Oral manifestations

L92.2 Granuloma faciale [eosinophilic granuloma of skin]
L92.2X   Face

L92.3 Foreign body granuloma of skin and subcutaneous tissue
L92.3X   Face

L93 Lupus erythematosus

Excludes: systemic lupus erythematosus (M32.–)

L93.0 Discoid lupus erythematosus
L93.0X   Oral manifestations

L94 Other localized connective tissue disorders

Excludes: systemic connective tissue disorders (M30–M35)

L94.0 Localized scleroderma [morphea]
L94.0X   Face

L94.1 Linear scleroderma
Includes: en coup de sabre lesion
L94.1X   Face

L98 Other disorders of skin and subcutaneous tissue, not elsewhere classified

L98.0 Pyogenic granuloma
L98.0X   Face

L98.8 Other specified disorders of skin and subcutaneous tissue
L98.80   Hereditary mucoepithelial dysplasia
L98.88   Other specified disorders of skin and subcutaneous
tissue, not elsewhere classified

CHAPTER XIII

Diseases of the musculoskeletal system and connective tissue

Arthropathies

Infectious arthropathies

M00 **Pyogenic arthritis**

M00.VX   Temporomandibular joint

M02 **Reactive arthropathies**

M02.3 **Reiter's disease**
M02.3X   Temporomandibular joint

Inflammatory polyarthropathies

M05 **Seropositive rheumatoid arthritis**

Includes: Felty's syndrome
M05.VX   Temporomandibular joint

M06 **Other rheumatoid arthritis**

M06.VX   Temporomandibular joint

M08 **Juvenile arthritis**

Includes: Still's disease
M08.VX   Temporomandibular joint

M12 **Other specific arthropathies**

M12.2 **Villonodular synovitis (pigmented)**
M12.2X   Temporomandibular joint

M12.5 **Traumatic arthropathy**
M12.5X   Temporomandibular joint

M13 Other arthritis

M13.9 **Arthritis, unspecified**
M13.9X Temporomandibular joint

Arthrosis

M15 Polyarthrosis

M15.VX Temporomandibular joint

M19 Other arthrosis

Includes: osteoarthritis
osteoarthrosis

M19.0 **Primary arthrosis of other joints**
M19.0X Temporomandibular joint

Systemic connective tissue disorders

M30 Polyarteritis nodosa and related conditions

M30.3 **Mucocutaneous lymph node syndrome [Kawasaki]**
M30.3X Oral manifestations

M31 Other necrotizing vasculopathies

M31.2 **Lethal midline granuloma**

M31.3 **Wegener's granulomatosis**
Includes: necrotizing respiratory granulomatosis
M31.3X Oral manifestations

M31.6 **Other giant cell arteritis**
M31.6X Oral manifestations

M32 Systemic lupus erythematosus

Excludes: discoid lupus erythematosus (L93.0)
M32.VX Oral manifestations

M33 Dermatopolymyositis

M33.VX Oral manifestations

M34 Systemic sclerosis

Includes: scleroderma
M34.VX Oral manifestations

M35 Other systemic invlovement of connective tissue

M35.0 Sicca syndrome [Sjögren]
M35.0X Oral manifestations

M35.2 Behçet's disease
M35.2X Oral manifestations

Soft tissue disorders

Disorders of muscles

M61 Calcification and ossification of muscle

Includes: myositis ossificans
M61.VX Head and neck

M62 Other disorders of muscle

M62.VX Head and neck

M72 Fibroblastic disorders

M72.3 Nodular fasciitis
M72.3X Head and neck

M72.4 Pseudosarcomatous fibromatosis
M72.4X Head and neck

M79 Other soft tissue disorders, not elsewhere classified

M79.1 Myalgia
Excludes: temporomandibular joint-pain-dysfunction syndrome
[Costen] (K07.60)
M79.1X Head and neck

M79.2 Neuralgia and neuritis, unspecified
M79.2X Head and neck

M79.5 Residual foreign body in soft tissue
Excludes: foreign body granuloma of skin and subcutaneous tissue
(L92.3)
M79.5X Head and neck

Osteopathies and chondropathies

Disorders of bone density and structure

M80 Osteoporosis with pathological fracture

M80.VX   Jaws

M81 Osteoporosis without pathological fracture

M81.VX   Jaws

M83 Adult osteomalacia

M83.VX   Jaws

M84 Disorders of continuity of bone

M84.0   **Malunion of fracture**
M84.0X   Head and neck

M84.1   **Nonunion of fracture [pseudarthrosis]**
M84.1X   Head and neck

M84.2   **Delayed union of fracture**
M84.2X   Head and neck

M84.4   **Pathological fracture, not elsewhere classified**
M84.4X   Head and neck

M85 Other disorders of bone density and structure

Excludes: aneurysmal bone cyst of jaw (K09.20)
fibrous dysplasia of jaw (K10.83)
osteogenesis imperfecta (Q78.0)
osteopetrosis (Q78.2)
osteopoikilosis (Q78.8)
polyostotic fibrous dysplasia (Q78.1)
solitary bone cyst of jaw (K09.21)

M85.2   **Hyperostosis of skull**

Other osteopathies

M88 Paget's disease of bone [osteitis deformans]

M88.0   **Paget's disease of skull**

M88.8 **Paget's disease of other bones**
M88.80   Maxilla
M88.81   Mandible
M88.88   Other facial bones

M88.9 **Paget's disease of bone, unspecified**

M89   Other disorders of bone

M89.8 **Other specified disorders of bone**
M89.80   Infantile cortical hyperostoses
M89.88   Other specified disorders of bone, not elsewhere classified

CHAPTER XIV

Diseases of the genitourinary system

Renal failure

N18   Chronic renal failure

N18.VX   Uraemia, oral manifestations

Noninflammatory disorders of female genital tract

N94   Pain and other conditions associated with female genital organs and menstrual cycle

N94.8   Other specified conditions associated with female genital organs and menstrual cycle
N94.8X   Oral manifestations
Gingivitis associated with menstrual cycle

N95   Menopausal and other perimenopausal disorders

N95.8   Other specified menopausal and perimenopausal disorders
N95.8X   Oral manifestations

CHAPTER XV

Pregnancy, childbirth and the puerperium

Other maternal disorders predominantly related to pregnancy

O21   **Excessive vomiting in pregnancy**

    O21.VX   Oral manifestations

O26   **Maternal care for other conditions predominantly related to pregnancy**

O26.8   **Other specified pregnancy-related conditions**
       O26.80   Pregnancy gingivitis
       O26.81   Pregnancy granuloma [granuloma gravidarum]
       O26.88   Other specified oral manifestations
       O26.89   Oral manifestation, unspecified

CHAPTER XVII

Congenital malformations, deformations and chromosomal abnormalities

Congenital malformations of the nervous system

Q07 **Other congenital malformations of nervous system**

> *Excludes:* neurofibromatosis (nonmalignant) (Q85.0)

Q07.8 **Other specified congenital malformations of nervous system**
Q07.8X   Jaw-winking syndrome [Marcus Gunn's syndrome]

Congenital malformations of eye, ear, face and neck

Q18 **Other congenital malformations of face and neck**

> *Excludes:* cleft lip and cleft palate (Q35–Q37)
> congenital malformations of skull and face bones (Q75.–)
> dentofacial anomalies [including malocclusion] (K07.–)
> malformation syndromes affecting facial appearance (Q87.0)

Q18.0 **Sinus, fistula and cyst of branchial cleft**

Q18.3 **Webbing of neck**
Pterygium colli

Q18.4 **Macrostomia**

Q18.5 **Microstomia**

Q18.6 **Macrocheilia**

Q18.7 **Microcheilia**

Q18.8 **Other specified congenital malformations of face and neck**

Q18.9 **Congenital malformation of face and neck, unspecified**

Congenital malformations of the circulatory system

Q21 Congenital malformations of cardiac septa

Q21.0   **Ventricular septal defect**
Q21.0X   Oral manifestations

Q21.1   **Atrial septal defect**
Q21.1X   Oral manifestations

Q21.3   **Tetralogy of Fallot**
Q21.3X   Oral manifestations

Q21.8   **Other congenital malformations of cardiac septa**
Q21.8X   Oral manifestations

Q21.9   **Congenital malformation of cardiac septum, unspecified**
Q21.9X   Oral manifestations

Q25 Congenital malformations of great arteries

Q25.0   **Patent ductus arteriosus**
Q25.0X   Oral manifestations

Q25.1   **Coarctation of aorta**
Q25.1X   Oral manifestations

Q27 Other congenital malformations of peripheral vascular system

Excludes: haemangioma and lymphangioma (D18.–)

Q27.3   **Peripheral arteriovenous malformation**
Includes: arteriovenous aneurysm of mandible
Q27.3X   Oral manifestations

Congenital malformations of the respiratory system

Q30 Congenital malformations of nose

Q30.8   **Other congenital malformations of nose**
Nose anomalies associated with jaw anomalies

Cleft lip and cleft palate

Excludes: Robin's syndrome (Q87.0)

Q35 Cleft palate

Includes: fissure of palate
palatoschisis
Excludes: cleft palate with cleft lip (Q37.–)

Q35.0 Cleft hard palate, bilateral

Q35.1 Cleft hard palate, unilateral
Cleft hard palate NOS

Q35.2 Cleft soft palate, bilateral

Q35.3 Cleft soft palate, unilateral
Cleft soft palate NOS

Q35.4 Cleft hard palate with cleft soft palate, bilateral

Q35.5 Cleft hard palate with cleft soft palate, unilateral
Cleft hard palate with cleft soft palate NOS

Q35.6 Cleft palate, medial

Q35.7 Cleft uvula

Q35.8 Cleft palate, unspecified, bilateral

Q35.9 Cleft palate, unspecified, unilateral
Cleft palate NOS

Q36 Cleft lip

Includes: cheiloschisis
congenital fissure of lip
harelip
labium leporinum
Excludes: cleft lip with cleft palate (Q37.–)

Q36.0 Cleft lip, bilateral

Q36.1 Cleft lip, medial

Q36.9 Cleft lip, unilateral
Cleft lip NOS

Q37 Cleft palate with cleft lip

Q37.0 Cleft hard palate with cleft lip, bilateral

Q37.1 **Cleft hard palate with cleft lip, unilateral**
Cleft hard palate with cleft lip NOS

Q37.2 **Cleft soft palate with cleft lip, bilateral**

Q37.3 **Cleft soft palate with cleft lip, unilateral**
Cleft soft palate with cleft lip NOS

Q37.4 **Cleft hard and soft palate with cleft lip, bilateral**

Q37.5 **Cleft hard and soft palate with cleft lip, unilateral**
Cleft hard and soft palate with cleft lip NOS

Q37.8 **Unspecified cleft palate with cleft lip, bilateral**

Q37.9 **Unspecified cleft palate with cleft lip, unilateral**
Cleft palate with cleft lip NOS

Other congenital malformations of the digestive system

Q38 Other congenital malformations of tongue, mouth and pharynx

Excludes: lingual tonsil (K14.88)
macrostomia (Q18.4)
median rhomboid glossitis (K14.2)
microstomia (Q18.5)
persistent thyroglossal or thyrolingual duct (Q89.20)
plicated tongue (K14.5)
thyroglossal cyst (Q89.21)
thyroglossal fistula (Q89.22)

Q38.0 **Congenital malformations of lips, not elsewhere classified**
Excludes: cleft lip (Q36.–)
• with cleft palate (Q37.–)
macrocheilia (Q18.6)
microcheilia (Q18.7)
Q38.00   Fistula of lip, congenital
Q38.01   Van der Woude's syndrome
Q38.08   Other congenital malformation of lip

Q38.1 **Ankyloglossia**
Tongue tie

Q38.2 **Macroglossia**

97

Q38.3 **Other congenital malformations of tongue**
Excludes: lingual thyroid (Q89.23)
persistent thyroglossal duct (Q89.20)
thyroglossal cyst (Q89.21)
thyroglossal fistula (Q89.22)
Q38.30 Aglossia
Q38.31 Bifid tongue
Q38.32 Adhesion of tongue, congenital
Q38.33 Fissure of tongue, congenital
Q38.34 Hypertrophy of tongue, congenital
Q38.35 Microglossia
Q38.36 Hypoplasia of tongue
Q38.38 Other specified congenital malformations of tongue
Q38.39 Congenital malformation of tongue, unspecified

Q38.4 **Congenital malformations of salivary glands and ducts**
Q38.40 Absence of salivary gland or duct
Q38.41 Accessory salivary gland or duct
Q38.42 Atresia of salivary gland or duct
Q38.43 Congenital fistula of salivary gland
Q38.48 Other specified congenital malformations of salivary glands and ducts
Q38.49 Congenital malformation of salivary glands and ducts, unspecified

Q38.5 **Congenital malformations of palate, not elsewhere classified**
Q38.50 Absence of uvula
Q38.51 High arched palate
Q38.58 Other congenital malformations of palate
Excludes: cleft palate (Q35.–)
• with cleft lip (Q37.–)

Q38.6 **Other congenital malformations of mouth**
Q38.60 Fordyce condition [Fordyce disease]
Q38.61 White sponge naevus [leukokeratosis oris]
Q38.68 Other specified congenital malformations of mouth
Q38.69 Congenital malformation of mouth, unspecified

Congenital malformations and deformations of the musculoskeletal system

Q67 Congenital musculoskeletal deformities of head, face, spine and chest

Excludes: congenital malformation syndromes classified to Q87.–

Q67.0 **Facial asymmetry**

Q67.1 **Compression facies**

Q67.2 **Dolichocephaly**

Q67.3 **Plagiocephaly**

Q67.4 **Other congenital deformities of skull, face and jaw**
Excludes: dentofacial anomalies [including malocclusion]
(K07.–)
Q67.40 Hemifacial atrophy
Q67.41 Hemifacial hypertrophy
Q67.48 Other specified congenital deformities of skull,
face and jaw
Q67.49 Congenital deformity of skull, face or jaw,
unspecified

Q68 Other congenital musculoskeletal deformities

Q68.0 **Congenital deformity of sternocleidomastoid muscle**
Q68.0X Congenital (sternomastoid) torticollis

Q75 Other congenital malformations of skull and face bones

Excludes: congenital malformation of face NOS (Q18.–)
congenital malformation syndromes classified to Q87.–
dentofacial anomalies [including malocclusion] (K07.–)
musculoskeletal deformities of head and face
(Q67.0–Q67.4)

Q75.0 **Craniosynostosis**
Q75.00 Acrocephaly
Q75.01 Imperfect fusion of skull
Q75.02 Oxycephaly
Q75.03 Trigonocephaly

Q75.1 **Craniofacial dysostosis**
Crouzon's disease

Q75.2 **Hypertelorism**

Q75.3 **Macrocephaly**

Q75.4 **Mandibulofacial dysostosis**

Q75.5 **Oculomandibular dysostosis**

Q75.8 **Other specified congenital malformations of skull and face bones**

Q75.9 **Congenital malformation of skull and face bones, unspecified**

Q76 Congenital malformations of spine and bony thorax

Q76.1 **Klippel–Feil syndrome**
Cervical fusion syndrome

Q77 Osteochondrodysplasia with defects of growth of tubular bones and spine

Excludes: mucopolysaccharidosis (E76.–)

Q77.4 **Achondroplasia**
Hypochondroplasia
Q77.4X   Oral manifestations

Q77.6 **Chondroectodermal dysplasia**
Ellis–van Creveld syndrome
Q77.6X   Oral manifestations

Q78 Other osteochondrodysplasias

Q78.0 **Osteogenesis imperfecta**
Includes: fragilitas ossium
Q78.0X   Oral manifestations

Q78.1 **Polyostotic fibrous dysplasia**
Includes: Albright(–McCune)(–Sternberg) syndrome
Q78.1X   Oral manifestations

Q78.2 **Osteopetrosis**
Includes: Albers–Schönberg syndrome
marble bone disease
Q78.2X   Oral manifestations

Q78.3 **Progressive diaphyseal dysplasia**
Q78.3X   Oral manifestations

Q78.8 **Other specified osteochondrodysplasias**
Includes: osteopoikilosis
Q78.8X   Oral manifestations

Q78.9 **Osteochondrodysplasia, unspecified**
Q78.9X   Oral manifestations

Q79 Congenital malformations of musculoskeletal system, not elsewhere classified

Excludes: congenital (sternomastoid) torticollis (Q68.0X)

Q79.6 Ehlers–Danlos syndrome
Q79.6X   Oral manifestations

Other congenital malformations

Q80 Congenital ichthyosis

Q80.VX   Oral manifestations

Q81 Epidermolysis bullosa

Q81.0 Epidermolysis bullosa simplex
Q81.0X   Oral manifestations

Q81.1 Epidermolysis bullosa letalis
Q81.1X   Oral manifestations

Q81.2 Epidermolysis bullosa dystrophica
Q81.2X   Oral manifestations

Q81.8 Other epidermolysis bullosa
Q81.8X   Oral manifestations

Q81.9 Epidermolysis bullosa, unspecified
Q81.9X   Oral manifestations

Q82 Other congenital malformations of skin

Excludes: acrodermatitis enteropathica (E83.2X)
congenital erythropoietic porphyria (E80.0)
Sturge–Weber(–Dimitri) syndrome (Q85.81)

Q82.1 Xeroderma pigmentosum
Q82.1X   Oral manifestations

Q82.2 Mastocytosis
Includes: urticaria pigmentosa
Q82.2X   Oral manifestations

Q82.3 Incontinentia pigmenti
Q82.3X   Oral manifestations

Q82.4   Ectodermal dysplasia (anhidrotic)
Excludes: Ellis–van Creveld syndrome (Q77.6)
Q82.4X   Oral manifestations

Q82.5   Congenital non-neoplastic naevus
Includes: naevus:
  • flammeus
  • portwine
  • sanguineous
  • strawberry
  • vascular NOS
  • verrucous
Excludes: café au lait spots (L81.3)
  lentigo (L81.4)
  naevus:
  • NOS (D22.–)
  • melanocytic (D22.–)
Q82.5X   Oral manifestations

Q82.8   Other specified congenital malformations of skin
Excludes: Ehlers–Danlos syndrome (Q79.6X)
Q82.80   Benign familial pemphigus [Hailey–Hailey]
Q82.81   Keratosis follicularis [Darier–White]
Q82.82   Inherited keratosis palmaris et plantaris
Q82.83   Dyskeratosis congenita
Q82.84   Pseudoxanthoma elasticum
Q82.85   Acrokeratosis verruciformis
Q82.88   Other

Q85   Phakomatoses, not elsewhere classified

Excludes: familial dysautonomia [Riley–Day] (G90.1)

Q85.0   Neurofibromatosis (nonmalignant)
Includes: von Recklinghausen's disease
Q85.0X   Oral manifestations

Q85.1   Tuberous sclerosis
Includes: Bourneville's disease
  epiloia
Q85.1X   Oral manifestations

Q85.8   Other phakomatoses, not elsewhere classified
Q85.80   Peutz–Jeghers syndrome
Q85.81   Sturge–Weber(–Dimitri) syndrome
Q85.88   Other specified phakomatoses

Q86 Congenital malformation syndromes due to known exogenous causes, not elsewhere classified

Q86.0 **Fetal alcohol syndrome (dysmorphic)**
Q86.0X Oral manifestations

Q87 Other specified congenital malformation syndromes affecting multiple systems

Q87.0 **Congenital malformation syndromes predominantly affecting facial appearance**
Q87.00 Acrocephalosyndactyly [Apert]
Q87.01 Goldenhar's syndrome
Q87.02 Moebius' syndrome
Q87.03 Oro-facial-digital syndrome
Q87.04 Treacher Collins syndrome
Q87.05 Robin's syndrome
Q87.08 Other

Q87.1 **Congenital malformation syndromes predominantly associated with short stature**
Includes: Noonan's syndrome
Excludes: Ellis–van Creveld syndrome (Q77.6)
Q87.1X Oral manifestations

Q87.2 **Congenital malformation syndromes predominantly involving limbs**
Q87.2X Oral manifestations

Q87.3 **Congenital malformation syndromes involving early overgrowth**
Q87.3X Oral manifestations

Q87.4 **Marfan's syndrome**
Q87.4X Oral manifestations

Q87.8 **Other specified congenital malformation syndromes, not elsewhere classified**
Q87.8X Oral manifestations

Q89 Other congenital malformations, not elsewhere classified

Q89.2 **Congenital malformations of other endocrine glands**
Q89.20 Persistent thyroglossal or thyrolingual duct
Q89.21 Thyroglossal cyst
Q89.22 Thyroglossal fistula

Q89.23 Lingual thyroid
Q89.28 Other specified congenital malformations of endocrine glands

Q89.8 **Other specified congenital malformations**

Chromosomal abnormalities, not elsewhere classified

Q90 Down's syndrome

Q90.VX Oral manifestations of Down's syndrome [trisomy 21]

Q91 Edwards' syndrome and Patau's syndrome

Q91.3X Oral manifestations of Edwards' syndrome [trisomy 18]
Q91.7X Oral manifestations of Patau's syndrome [trisomy 13]

Q93 Monosomies and deletions from the autosomes, not elsewhere classified

Q93.3 **Deletion of short arm of chromosome 4**
Includes: Wolff–Hirschorn syndrome
Q93.3X Oral manifestations

Q93.4 **Deletion of short arm of chromosome 5**
Includes: cri-du-chat syndrome
Q93.4X Oral manifestations

Q96 Turner's syndrome

Excludes: Noonan's syndrome (Q87.1)
Q96.VX Oral manifestations

Q98 Other sex chromosome abnormalities, male phenotype, not elsewhere classified

Q98.V0 Klinefelter's syndrome, oral manifestations
Q98.V1 Oral manifestations of other sex chromosome abnormalities, male phenotype

Q99 Other chromosome abnormalities, not elsewhere classified

Q99.2 **Fragile X chromosome**
Q99.2X Oral manifestations

Symptoms, signs and abnormal clinical and laboratory findings, not elsewhere classified

This chapter includes symptoms, signs, abnormal results of clinical or other investigative procedures, and ill-defined conditions regarding which no diagnosis classifiable elsewhere is recorded.

Symptoms and signs involving the circulatory and respiratory systems

R04 **Haemorrhage from respiratory passages**

R04.0 **Epistaxis**

R04.1 **Haemorrhage from throat**

R06 **Abnormalities of breathing**

R06.5 **Mouth breathing**
Snoring
Excludes: dry mouth NOS (R68.2)

R07 **Pain in throat and chest**

Excludes: dysphagia (R13)

R07.0 **Pain in throat**

Symptoms and signs involving the digestive system and abdomen

R13 **Dysphagia**

R17 **Unspecified jaundice**

R17.XX   Oral manifestations

R19   Other symptoms and signs involving the digestive system and abdomen

R19.6   Halitosis

Symptoms and signs involving the skin and subcutaneous tissue

R20   Disturbances of skin sensation

R20.0   Anaesthesia of skin

R20.1   Hypoaesthesia of skin

R20.2   Paraesthesia of skin

R20.3   Hyperaesthesia

R20.8   Other and unspecified disturbances of skin sensation

R22   Localized swelling, mass and lump of skin and subcutaneous tissue

Includes: subcutaneous nodules (localized) (superficial)
Excludes: enlarged lymph nodes NOS (R59.–)

R22.0   Localized swelling, mass and lump, head

R22.1   Localized swelling, mass and lump, neck

R23   Other skin changes

R23.0   Cyanosis
R23.0X   Oral manifestations

R23.3   Flushing
Excessive blushing

R23.3   Spontaneous ecchymoses
Includes: petechiae
R23.3X   Oral manifestations

Symptoms and signs involving the nervous and musculoskeletal systems

R25 Abnormal involuntary movements

R25.0 Abnormal head movements

R25.3 Fasciculation
Twitching NOS

Symptoms and signs involving cognition, perception, emotional state and behaviour

R43 Disturbances of smell and taste

R43.2 Parageusia

R43.8 Other and unspecified disturbances of smell and taste

Symptoms and signs involving speech and voice

R47 Speech disturbances, not elsewhere classified

Excludes: specific developmental disorders of speech and language (F80. –)

R47.0 Dysphasia and aphasia

General symptoms and signs

R51 Headache

Excludes: atypical facial pain (G50.1)
migraine (G43.VX)
trigeminal neuralgia (G50.0)
R51.X0 Headache, unspecified
R51.X1 Facial pain, unspecified

R59 Enlarged lymph nodes

Includes: swollen glands
Excludes: lymphadenitis (I88.–, L04.–)
R59.VX Head and neck

R68 Other general symptoms and signs

R68.2 **Dry mouth, unspecified**
Excludes: due to:
- salivary gland hyposecretion (K11.70)
- sicca syndrome [Sjögren] (M35.0)

Abnormal findings on examination of other body fluids, substances and tissues without diagnosis

R85 Abnormal findings in specimens from digestive organs and abdominal cavity

R85.XX   Abnormal findings in saliva

Abnormal findings on diagnostic imaging and in function studies, without diagnosis

R93 Abnormal findings on diagnostic imaging of other body structures

R93.0 **Abnormal findings on diagnostic imaging of skull and head, not elsewhere classified**

CHAPTER XIX

Injury, poisoning and certain other consequences of external causes

Where multiple sites of injury are specified in the titles, the word "with" indicates involvement of both sites, and the word "and" indicates involvement of either or both sites.

The principle of multiple coding of injuries should be followed wherever possible. Combination categories for multiple injuries are provided for use when there is insufficient detail as to the nature of the individual conditions, or for primary tabulation purposes when it is more convenient to record a single code; otherwise, the component injuries should be coded separately. Reference should also be made to morbidity or mortality rules and guidelines (see ICD-10, Volume 2).

The body region-related blocks given here contain injuries at the three-character level classified by type as listed below:

Superficial injury including:
abrasion
blister (nonthermal)
contusion, including bruise and haematoma
injury from superficial foreign body (splinter) without major open wound
insect bite (nonvenomous)

Open wound including:
animal bite
cut
laceration
puncture wound:
• NOS
• with (penetrating) foreign body

Fracture including:
Fracture:
• closed:

- comminuted ⎫
- depressed ⎪
- elevated ⎪
- fissured ⎪
- greenstick ⎬ with or without delayed healing
- impacted ⎪
- linear ⎪
- simple ⎪
- spiral ⎭
• dislocated
• displaced
• open:
   - compound ⎫
   - infected ⎪
   - missile ⎬ with or without delayed healing
   - puncture ⎪
   - with foreign body ⎭

Excludes: fracture:
       • pathological (M84.4)
         • with osteoporosis (M80.–)
       • stress (M84.3)
       malunion of fracture (M84.0)
       nonunion of fracture [pseudarthrosis] (M84.1)

Dislocation, sprain and strain including:
avulsion ⎫
laceration ⎪
sprain ⎪
strain ⎪   ⎧joint (capsule)
traumatic: ⎬ of ⎨
• haemarthrosis ⎪   ⎩ligament
• rupture ⎪
• subluxation ⎪
• tear ⎭

Injury to nerves including:
traumatic:
• division of nerve
• paralysis (transient)

Injury to blood vessels including

avulsion
cut
laceration
traumatic:
• aneurysm or fistula
  (arteriovenous)
• arterial haematoma
• rupture

} of blood vessels

Injury to muscle and tendon including

avulsion
cut
laceration
traumatic rupture

} of muscle and tendon

Crushing injury

Other and unspecified injuries

Injuries to the head

Includes: injuries of:
  • ear
  • eye
  • face [any part]
  • gum (gingiva, alveolar ridge)
  • jaw
  • mandibular joint area
  • oral cavity
  • palate
  • periocular area
  • scalp
  • tongue
  • tooth

Excludes: burns and corrosions (T20–T32)
        effects of foreign body:
          • in:
            • ear (T16)
            • larynx (T17.3)
            • mouth NOS (T18.0)

- nose (T17.0–T17.1)
- pharynx (T17.2)
- on external eye (T15.–)
frostbite (T33–T35)
insect bite or sting, venomous (T63.4)

S00 Superficial injury of head

Excludes: cerebral contusion (diffuse) (S06. 2)
- focal (S06.3)
injury of eye and orbit (S05.–)

S00.0 Superficial injury of scalp

S00.1 Contusion of eyelid and periocular area
Black eye

S00.2 Other superficial injuries of eyelid and periocular area

S00.3 Superficial injury of nose

S00.4 Superficial injury of ear

S00.5 Superficial injury of lip and oral cavity
S00.50 Superficial injury of internal cheek
S00.51 Superficial injury of other parts of mouth (including tongue)
S00.52 Superficial injury of lip
S00.59 Superficial injury of lip and oral cavity, unspecified

S00.7 Multiple superficial injuries of head

S00.8 Superficial injury of other parts of head

S00.9 Superficial injury of head, part unspecified

S01 Open wound of head

S01.0 Open wound of scalp
Excludes: avulsion of scalp (S08.0)

S01.1 Open wound of eyelid and periocular area
Open wound of eyelid and periocular area with or without involvement of lacrimal passages

S01.2 Open wound of nose

S01.3 Open wound of ear

S01.4 Open wound of cheek and temporomandibular area
S01.40 Open wound of cheek
S01.41 Open wound of temporomandibular area

S01.5 Open wound of lip and oral cavity
Excludes: cheek (S01.40)
        tooth:
        • dislocation (S03.2)
        • fracture (S02.5)
S01.50 Open wound of mouth (including tongue)
S01.51 Open wound of lip
S01.59 Open wound of lip and oral cavity, unspecified

S01.7 Multiple open wounds of head

S01.8 Open wound of other parts of head

S01.9 Open wound of head, part unspecified

S02 Fracture of skull and facial bones

Note: For primary coding of fracture of skull and facial bones with associated intracranial injury, reference should be made to the morbidity or mortality coding rules and guidelines (see ICD-10, Volume 2).

Where it is not possible or not desired to use multiple coding to identify fracture and open wound, 0 (closed) or 1 (open) may be used in the sixth character position, X being added in the fifth character position if no fifth character is given. A fracture not indicated as closed or open should be classified as closed.

S02.0 Fracture of vault of skull
Frontal bone
Parietal bone

S02.1 Fracture of base of skull
Fossa:
• anterior
• middle
• posterior
Occiput
Orbital roof
Sinus:
• ethmoid
• frontal
Sphenoid
Temporal bone

Excludes: orbit NOS (S02.8)
orbital floor (S02.3)

S02.2   Fracture of nasal bones

S02.3   Fracture of orbital floor
Excludes: orbit NOS (S02.8)
orbital roof (S02.1)

S02.4   Fracture of malar and maxillary bones
S02.40   Fracture of maxillary alveolar process
S02.41   Fracture of malar bone [zygoma]
S02.42   Fracture of maxilla
S02.47   Multiple fractures of malar and maxillary bones

S02.5   Fracture of tooth
Includes: primary (deciduous) and permanent teeth
S02.50   Fracture of enamel of tooth only
Enamel chipping
S02.51   Fracture of crown of tooth without pulpal
involvement
S02.52   Fracture of crown of tooth with pulpal involvement
S02.53   Fracture of root of tooth
S02.54   Fracture of crown with root of tooth
S02.57   Multiple fractures of teeth
S02.59   Fracture of tooth, unspecified

S02.6   Fracture of mandible
S02.60   Fracture of alveolar process
S02.61   Fracture of body of mandible
S02.62   Fracture of condyle
S02.63   Fracture of coronoid process
S02.64   Fracture of ramus
S02.65   Fracture of symphysis
S02.66   Fracture of angle
S02.67   Multiple fractures of mandible
S02.69   Fracture of mandible, part unspecified

S02.7   Multiple fractures involving skull and facial bones
S02.70   Without (mention of) intracranial injury
S02.71   With (mention of) intracranial injury

S02.8   Fractures of other skull and facial bones
Alveolus
Orbit NOS
Palate
Excludes: orbital:
- floor (S02.3)
- roof (S02.1)

S02.9   Fracture of skull and facial bones, part unspecified

S03   Dislocation, sprain and strain of joints and ligaments of head

S03.0   Dislocation of jaw
Excludes: recurrent subluxation of temporomandibular joint
(K07.62)

S03.1   Dislocation of septal cartilage of nose

S03.2   Dislocation of tooth
S03.20   Luxation of tooth
S03.21   Intrusion or extrusion of tooth
S03.22   Avulsion of tooth [exarticulation]

S03.3   Dislocation of other and unspecified parts of head

S03.4   Sprain and strain of jaw
Temporomandibular (joint) (ligament)

S04   Injury of cranial nerves

S04.3   Injury of trigeminal nerve
Fifth cranial nerve

S04.5   Injury of facial nerve
Seventh cranial nerve

S04.8   Injury of other cranial nerves
S04.80   Injury of glossopharyngeal [9th cranial] nerve
S04.81   Injury of hypoglossal [12th cranial] nerve

S04.9   Injury of unspecified cranial nerve

S07   Crushing injury of head

S07.0   Crushing injury of face

S07.1   Crushing injury of skull

S07.8   Crushing injury of other parts of head

S07.9   Crushing injury of head, part unspecified

S09   Other and unspecified injuries of head

S09.0   Injury of blood vessels of head, not elsewhere classified

115

S09.1 **Injury of muscle and tendon of head**

S09.7 **Multiple injuries of head**

S09.8 **Other specified injuries of head**

S09.9 **Unspecified injury of head**
Injury of:
• ear NOS
• face NOS
• nose NOS

Injuries to the neck

Includes: injuries of
• supraclavicular region
• throat
Excludes: burns and corrosions (T20.–, T28.–)

S10 Superficial injury of neck

S11 Open wound of neck

S15 Injury of blood vessels at neck level

S15.0 **Injury of carotid artery**
Carotid artery (common) (external) (internal)

S15.2 **Injury of external jugular vein**

S15.3 **Injury of internal jugular vein**

S15.7 **Injury of multiple blood vessels at neck level**

S15.8 **Injury of other blood vessels at neck level**

S15.9 **Injury of unspecified blood vessel at neck level**

Injuries involving multiple body regions

Excludes: burns and corrosions (T20.–, T28.–)
frostbite (T33–T35)
insect bite, venomous (T63.4)
multiple injuries involving only one body region — see S-section

T00 Superficial injuries involving multiple body regions

T00.0 Superficial injuries involving head with neck
Superficial injuries of sites classifiable to S00.– and S10

T01 Open wounds involving multiple body regions

T01.0 Open wounds involving head with neck
Open wounds of sites classifiable to S01.– and S11

T02 Fractures involving multiple body regions

[See note under S02.–]

T02.0 Fractures involving head with neck

T03 Dislocations, sprains and strains involving multiple body regions

T03.0 Dislocations, sprains and strains involving head with neck

T04 Crushing injuries involving multiple body regions

T04.0 Crushing injuries involving head with neck

Effects of foreign body entering through natural orifice

Excludes: foreign body:
- accidentally left in operation wound (T81.5)
- in penetrating wound—see open wound by body region
- residual, in soft tissue (M79.5)
splinter without major open wound—see superficial injury by
   body region

T17 Foreign body in respiratory tract

T18 Foreign body in alimentary tract

T18.0 Foreign body in mouth

Burns and corrosions

Includes: burns (thermal) from:
- electrical heating appliances
- electricity
- flame
- friction
- hot air and hot gases
- hot objects
- lightning
- radiation

chemical burns [corrosions] (external) (internal)

scalds

Burns and corrosions of external body surface, specified by site

Includes: burns and corrosions of:
- first degree [erythema]
- second degree [blisters] [epidermal loss]
- third degree [deep necrosis of underlying tissue] [full-thickness skin loss]

T20   Burn and corrosion of head and neck

> *Includes:*   ear [any part]
> eye with other parts of face, head and neck
> lip
> nose (septum)
> scalp [any part]
> temple (region)
>
> *Excludes:* burn and corrosion of mouth and pharynx (T28.–)

T20.0   **Burn of unspecified degree of head and neck**

T20.1   **Burn of first degree of head and neck**

T20.2   **Burn of second degree of head and neck**

T20.3   **Burn of third degree of head and neck**

T20.4   **Corrosion of unspecified degree of head and neck**

T20.5   **Corrosion of first degree of head and neck**

T20.6   **Corrosion of second degree of head and neck**

T20.7   **Corrosion of third degree of head and neck**

T28   Burn and corrosion of other internal organs

T28.0   **Burn of mouth and pharynx**

T28.5   **Corrosion of mouth and pharynx**

Frostbite

T33   Superficial frostbite

Includes: frostbite with partial-thickness skin loss
Excludes: superficial frostbite involving multiple body regions
(T35.0)

T33.0   **Superficial frostbite of head**

T33.1   **Superficial frostbite of neck**

T34   Frostbite with tissue necrosis

Excludes: frostbite with tissue necrosis involving multiple body
regions (T35.1)

T34.0   **Frostbite with tissue necrosis of head**

T34.1   **Frostbite with tissue necrosis of neck**

T35   Frostbite involving multiple body regions and unspecified frostbite

T35.0   **Superficial frostbite involving multiple body regions**

T35.1   **Frostbite with tissue necrosis involving multiple body regions**

T35.2   **Unspecified frostbite of head and neck**

Poisoning by drugs, medicaments and biological substances

Includes: overdose of these substances
wrong substance given or taken in error
Excludes: adverse effects ["hypersensitivity", "reaction", etc.] of correct
substance properly administered; such cases are to be classified
according to the nature of the adverse effect

T36 Poisoning by systemic antibiotics

Excludes: antibiotics, locally applied NEC (T49.0)

T37 Poisoning by other systemic anti-infectives and antiparasitics

Excludes: anti-infectives, locally applied NEC (T49.0)

T38 Poisoning by hormones and their synthetic substitutes and antagonists, not elsewhere classified

Excludes: mineralocorticoids and their antagonists (T50)
　　　　　oxytocic hormones (T48)
　　　　　parathyroid hormones and derivatives (T50)

T39 Poisoning by nonopioid analgesics, antipyretics and antirheumatics

T40 Poisoning by narcotics and psychodysleptics [hallucinogens]

Excludes: drug dependence and related mental and behavioural disorders due to psychoactive substance use (F10–F19)

T41　Poisoning by anaesthetics and therapeutic gases

Excludes: benzodiazepines (T42.4)
　　　　　cocaine (T40.5)
　　　　　opioids (T40.0–T40.2)

T42 Poisoning by antiepileptic, sedative–hypnotic and antiparkinsonism drugs

Excludes: drug dependence and related mental and behavioural disorders due to psychoactive substance use (F10–F19)

T43 Poisoning by psychotropic drugs, not elsewhere classified

Excludes: appetite depressants (T50)
　　　　　barbiturates (T42)

benzodiazepines (T42)
drug dependence and related mental and behavioural
    disorders due to psychoactive substance use (F10–F19)
methaqualone (T42)
psychodysleptics [hallucinogens] (T40)

T44 Poisoning by drugs primarily affecting the autonomic nervous system

T45 Poisoning by primarily systemic and haematological agents, not elsewhere classified

T46 Poisoning by agents primarily affecting the cardiovascular system

Excludes: metaraminol (T44)

T47 Poisoning by agents primarily affecting the gastrointestinal system

T48 Poisoning by agents primarily acting on smooth and skeletal muscles and the respiratory system

T49 Poisoning by topical agents primarily affecting skin and mucous membrane and by ophthalmological, otorhinolaryngological and dental drugs

T49.0 Local antifungal, anti-infective and anti-inflammatory drugs, not elsewhere classified

T49.7 Dental drugs, topically applied

T50 Poisoning by diuretics and other and unspecified drugs, medicaments and biological substances

Toxic effects of substances chiefly nonmedicinal as to source

Excludes: corrosions (T20.–, T28.–)
localized toxic effects classified elsewhere (A00–R99)

T51 **Toxic effect of alcohol**

T52 **Toxic effect of organic solvents**

T53 **Toxic effect of halogen derivatives of aliphatic and aromatic hydrocarbons**

T54 **Toxic effect of corrosive substances**

T55 **Toxic effect of soaps and detergents**

T56 **Toxic effect of metals**

Includes: fumes and vapours of metals
metals from all sources, except medicinal substances
Excludes: arsenic and its compounds (T57.0)
manganese and its compounds (T57.–)
thallium (T60)

T56.0 **Lead and its compounds**

T56.1 **Mercury and its compounds**
Acrodynia

T57 **Toxic effect of other inorganic substances**

T57.0 **Arsenic and its compounds**

T58 **Toxic effect of carbon monoxide**

From all sources

T59 **Toxic effect of other gases, fumes and vapours**

Aerosol propellants
Excludes: chlorofluorocarbons (T53)

T60 Toxic effect of pesticides

Wood preservatives

T61 Toxic effect of noxious substances eaten as seafood

T62 Toxic effect of other noxious substances eaten as food

T65 Toxic effect of other and unspecified substances

T65.2 Tobacco and nicotine

Other and unspecified effects of external causes

T66 Unspecified effects of radiation

Radiation sickness
Excludes: specified adverse effects of radiation, such as:
• burns (T21.–, T28.–)
• related disorders of the skin and subcutaneous tissue (L56.–)

T67 Effects of heat and light

Excludes: burns (T21.–, T28.–)
radiation-related disorders of skin and subcutaneous tissue (L56.–)

T70 Effects of air pressure and water pressure

T70.1 Sinus barotrauma

Effects of change in ambient atmospheric pressure on sinuses

T70.2 Other and unspecified effects of high altitude

Aerodontalgia

T70.3 Caisson disease [decompression sickness]

T78   Adverse effects, not elsewhere classified

> *Note:*   This category is to be used as the primary code to identify
> the effects, not elsewhere classifiable, of unknown, un-
> determined or ill-defined causes. For multiple coding pur-
> poses this category may be used as an additional code to
> identify the effects of conditions classified elsewhere.
>
> *Excludes:* complications of surgical and medical care NEC
> (T80–T88)

T78.3   Angioneurotic oedema
Giant urticaria
Quincke's oedema
Excludes: urticaria (L50.–)
• serum (T80.6)

T78.4   Allergy, unspecified
Allergic reaction NOS
Hypersensitivity NOS
Idiosyncrasy NOS
Excludes: allergic reaction NOS to correct medicinal substance
properly administered (T88)

Complications of surgical and medical care, not elsewhere classified

Use additional external cause code (Chapter XX), if desired, to identify devices
involved and details of circumstances.

Use additional code (B95–B97), if desired, to identify infectious agent.

Excludes: adverse effects of drugs and medicaments (A00–R99, T78.–)
burns and corrosions from local applications and irradiation
(T21.–, T28.–)
poisoning and toxic effects of drugs and chemicals (T36, T62,
T65.–)
specified complications classified elsewhere

T80   Complications following infusion, transfusion and therapeutic injection

T81 Complications of procedures, not elsewhere classified

Excludes: adverse effect of drug NOS (T88.7)
    specified complications classified elsewhere, such as
    complications of prosthetic devices, implants and grafts
    (T82–T85)

T81.0 **Haemorrhage and haematoma complicating a procedure, not elsewhere classified**

T81.1 **Shock during or resulting from a procedure, not elsewhere classified**

Collapse NOS
Shock (endotoxic) (hypovolaemic) (septic) } during or following a procedure
Postoperative shock NOS

Excludes: shock:
- anaesthetic (T88)
- anaphylactic, due to:
  - correct medicinal substance properly administered (T88)
  - serum (T80)

T81.2 **Accidental puncture and laceration during a procedure, not elsewhere classified**

Accidental perforation of:

- blood vessel
- nerve } by { catheter / endoscope / instrument / probe } during a procedure
- organ

T81.3 **Disruption of operation wound, not elsewhere classifed**

Dehiscence
Rupture } of operation wound

T81.4 **Infection following a procedure, not elsewhere classified**

Abscess:
- stitch
- wound } postprocedural
Septicaemia

Excludes: infection due to prosthetic devices, implants and grafts (T84.5–T84.7, T85.7)

T81.5   **Foreign body accidentally left in body cavity or operation wound following a procedure**
Excludes: obstruction or perforation due to prosthetic devices and implants intentionally left in body (T84.0–T84.4)
  T81.50   Amalgam tattoo
  T81.58   Other
  T81.59   Unspecified

T81.8   **Other complications of procedures, not elsewhere classified**
Emphysema (subcutaneous) resulting from a procedure
Persistent postoperative fistula

T84   Complications of internal orthopaedic prosthetic devices, implants and grafts

Excludes: failure and rejection of transplanted organs or tissues (T86. –)

T84.0   **Mechanical complication of internal joint prosthesis**

T84.2   **Mechanical complication of internal fixation device of other bones**

T84.3   **Mechanical complication of other bone devices, implants and grafts**

T84.4   **Mechanical complication of other internal orthopaedic devices, implants and grafts**

T84.5   **Infection and inflammatory reaction due to internal joint prosthesis**

T84.6   **Infection and inflammatory reaction due to internal fixation device [any site]**

T84.7   **Infection and inflammatory reaction due to other internal orthopaedic prosthetic devices, implants and grafts**

T84.8   **Other complications of internal orthopaedic prosthetic devices, implants and grafts**

T84.9   **Unspecified complication of internal orthopaedic prosthetic device, implant and graft**

T86   Failure and rejection of transplanted organs and tissues

T86.0   **Bone-marrow transplant rejection**

T86.8 **Failure and rejection of other transplanted organs and tissues**
Transplant failure or rejection of
- bone
- skin (allograft) (autograft)
- tooth

T88 Other complications of surgical and medical care, not elsewhere classified

Sequelae of injuries, of poisoning and of other consequences of external causes

Note: These categories are to be used to indicate conditions in S00–S99 and T00–T88 as the cause of late effects, which are themselves classified elsewhere. The "sequelae" include those specified as such, or as late effects, and those present one year or more after the acute injury.

T90 Sequelae of injuries of head

T91 Sequelae of injuries of neck and trunk

T95 Sequelae of burns, corrosions and frostbite

T95.0 **Sequelae of burn, corrosion and frostbite of head and neck**
Sequelae of injury classifiable to T20.–, T33.0–T33.1,
T34.0–T34.1 and T35.2

CHAPTER XX

External causes of morbidity and mortality

Intentional self-harm

X62   **Intentional self-poisoning by and exposure to narcotics and psychodysleptics [hallucinogens], not elsewhere classified**

    X62.VX   Cocaine, oral manifestations

X77   **Intentional self-harm by steam, hot vapours and hot objects**

    X77.VX   Oral manifestations

Complications of medical and surgical care

Drugs, medicaments and biological substances causing adverse effects in therapeutic use

Y40   **Systemic antibiotics**

    Excludes: antibiotics, topically used (Y56.–)
                 antineoplastic antibiotics (Y43.3)

Y40.0   **Penicillins**
    Y40.0X   Oral manifestations

Y40.2   **Chloramphenicol group**
    Y40.2X   Oral manifestations

Y40.3   **Macrolides**
    Includes: erythromycin
    Y40.3X   Oral manifestations

Y40.4   **Tetracyclines**
    Y40.4X   Oral manifestations

Y40.7 **Antifungal antibiotics, systemically used**
Y40.7X   Oral manifestations

Y40.8 **Other systemic antibiotics**
Y40.8X   Oral manifestations

Y40.9 **Systemic antibiotic, unspecified**
Y40.9X   Oral manifestations

Y41 Other systemic anti-infectives and antiparasitics

Y41.0 **Sulfonamides**
Y41.0X   Oral manifestations

Y41.2 **Antimalarials and drugs acting on other blood protozoa**
Y41.2X   Oral manifestations

Y41.5 **Antiviral drugs**
Y41.5X   Oral manifestations

Y41.9 **Systemic anti-infective and antiparasitic, unspecified**
Y41.9X   Oral manifestations

Y42 Hormones and their synthetic substitutes and antagonists, not elsewhere classified

Y42.4 **Oral contraceptives**
Y42.4X   Oral manifestations

Y42.9 **Other and unspecified hormone antagonists**
Y42.9X   Oral manifestations

Y43 Primarily systemic agents

Y43.3 **Other antineoplastic drugs**
Y43.3X   Oral manifestations

Y43.4 **Immunosuppressive agents**
Y43.4X   Oral manifestations

Y43.9 **Primarily systemic agent, unspecified**
Y43.9X   Oral manifestations

Y45 Analgesics, antipyretics and anti-inflammatory drugs

Y45.0 **Opioids and related analgesics**
Y45.0X   Oral manifestations

Y45.1 **Salicylates**
Y45.1X   Oral manifestations

Y45.3 **Other nonsteroidal anti-inflammatory drugs (NSAID)**
Y45.3X   Oral manifestations

Y45.4 **Antirheumatics**
Y45.4X   Oral manifestations

Y45.9 **Analgesic, antipyretic and anti-inflammatory drug, unspecified**
Y45.9X   Oral manifestations

Y46 **Antiepileptics and antiparkinsonism drugs**

Y46.2 **Hydantoin derivatives**
Y46.2X   Oral manifestations

Y48 **Anaesthetics and therapeutic gases**

Y48.0 **Inhaled anaesthetics**
Y48.0X   Oral manifestations

Y48.3 **Local anaesthetics**
Y48.3X   Oral manifestations

Y48.4 **Anaesthetic, unspecified**
Y48.4X   Oral manifestations

Y49 **Psychotropic drugs, not elsewhere classified**

Y49.9 **Psychotropic drug, unspecified**
Y49.9X   Oral manifestations

Y52 **Agents primarily affecting the cardiovascular system**

Y52.1 **Calcium-channel blockers**
Y52.1X   Oral manifestations

Y56 **Topical agents primarily affecting skin and mucous membrane and ophthalmological, otorhinolaryngological and dental drugs**

Y56.0 **Local antifungal, anti-infective and anti-inflammatory drugs, not elsewhere classified**
Y56.0X   Oral manifestations

Y56.7 **Dental drugs, topically applied**
Y56.7X   Oral manifestations

Misadventures to patients during surgical and medical care

Y60 **Unintentional cut, puncture, perforation or haemorrhage during surgical and medical care**

Y60.0 During surgical operation

Y61 **Foreign object accidentally left in body during surgical and medical care**

Y61.0 During surgical operation

Y65 **Other misadventures during surgical and medical care**

Y65.8 Other specified misadventures during surgical and medical care

Medical devices associated with adverse incidents in diagnostic and therapeutic use

Y82 **Other and unspecified medical devices associated with adverse incidents**

Y82.2 Prosthetic and other implants, materials and accessory devices

Y82.3 Surgical instruments, materials and devices (including sutures)

Y82.8 Miscellaneous devices, not elsewhere classified

Extract from numerical index of morphology of neoplasms (ICD-O)

In Chapter II, the ICD-DA—like ICD-10—provides for the coding of neoplasms. The classification is mainly on an anatomical (topographical) basis, although there are main subdivisions into malignant, benign, uncertain behaviour, etc. However, with few exceptions, Chapter II does not allow for a precise histopathological (morphological) coding of the tumour type.

The World Health Organization has published an adaptation and extension of Chapter II of ICD-10 under the title *International Classification of Diseases for Oncology*[1] (ICD-O), which gives a dual-axis classification, providing coding systems for morphology as well as for topography. Those users who require a precise histopathological coding should refer to that volume. For convenience, however, an extract of the relevant part of the morphology (M) code of the ICD-O is included here, giving the coding for the primary and metastatic tumours most likely to be found in the mouth and jaws. It must be emphasized that this is only an extract; for example, in the section relating to lymphomas, ICD-O provides a detailed subdivision if this is required.

The morphology code numbers consist of five digits; the first four identify the histological type of the neoplasm and the fifth, following a slash or solidus, indicates its behaviour. The one-digit behaviour code is as follows:

/0   Benign

/1   Uncertain whether benign or malignant
Borderline malignancy
Low malignant potential

/2   Carcinoma in situ
Intraepithelial
Noninfiltrating
Noninvasive

---

[1] *International Classification of Diseases for Oncology*, 2nd ed. Geneva, World Health Organization, 1990.

/3 Malignant, primary site

/6 Malignant, metastatic site
Malignant, secondary site

/9 Malignant, uncertain whether primary or metastatic site
The ICD-O behaviour digit /9 is not applicable in the ICD context, since all malignant neoplasms are presumed to be primary (/3) or secondary (/6), according to other information on the medical record.

Coded nomenclature for morphology of neoplasms

M800 Neoplasms NOS
M8000/0   Neoplasm, benign
                Tumour, benign
M8000/1   Neoplasm, uncertain whether benign or malignant
                Neoplasm NOS
                Tumour NOS
M8000/3   Neoplasm, malignant
                Tumour, malignant
                Malignancy
                Cancer
M8000/6   Neoplasm, metastatic
                Tumour, metastatic
                Tumour, embolus
M8001/0   Tumour cells, benign
M8001/1   Tumour cells, uncertain whether benign or malignant
M8001/3   Tumour cells, malignant

M801–M804 Epithelial neoplasms NOS
M8010/0   Epithelial tumour, benign
M8010/2   Carcinoma in situ NOS
                Intraepithelial carcinoma NOS
M8010/3   Carcinoma NOS
                Epithelial tumour, malignant
M8010/6   Carcinoma, NOS, metastatic
                Secondary carcinoma
M8011/3   Epithelioma, malignant
                Epithelioma, NOS
M8020/3   Undifferentiated carcinoma, NOS
M8021/3   Anaplastic carcinoma, NOS
M8022/3   Pleomorphic carcinoma
M8032/3   Spindle cell carcinoma
M8033/3   Pseudosarcomatous carcinoma

M8041/3   Small cell carcinoma, NOS
          Round cell carcinoma
M8042/3   Oat cell carcinoma

M805–M808   Squamous cell neoplasms
M8050/0   Papilloma NOS
M8050/3   Papillary carcinoma, NOS
M8051/0   Verrucous papilloma
M8051/3   Verrucous carcinoma
M8052/0   Squamous cell papilloma
          Squamous papilloma
          Keratotic papilloma
M8052/3   Papillary squamous cell carcinoma
M8053/0   Inverted papilloma
M8060/0   Papillomatosis NOS
M8070/2   Squamous cell carcinoma in situ NOS
          Epidermoid carcinoma in situ NOS
          Intraepidermal carcinoma NOS
          Intraepithelial squamous cell carcinoma
M8070/3   Squamous cell carcinoma NOS
          Epidermoid carcinoma NOS
          Squamous carcinoma
M8070/6   Squamous cell carcinoma, metastatic NOS
M8071/3   Squamous cell carcinoma, keratinizing NOS
M8074/3   Squamous cell carcinoma, spindle cell
M8075/3   Squamous cell carcinoma, adenoid type
M8076/2   Squamous cell carcinoma in situ with questionable stromal
          invasion
          Epidermoid carcinoma in situ with questionable stromal
            invasion
M8076/3   Squamous cell carcinoma, microinvasive
M8080/2   Queyrat's erythroplasia
M8081/2   Bowen's disease
          Intraepidermal squamous cell carcinoma, Bowen's type
M8082/3   Lymphoepithelial carcinoma
          Lymphoepithelioma

M809–M811   Basal cell neoplasms
M8090/1   Basal cell tumour NOS
M8090/3   Basal cell carcinoma NOS
          Basal cell epithelioma
M8091/3   Multicentric basal cell carcinoma
M8094/3   Basosquamous carcinoma

M812–M813   Transitional cell papillomas and carcinomas
M8122/3   Transitional cell carcinoma, spindle cell type

M814–M838   Adenomas and adenocarcinomas
M8140/0   Adenoma NOS
M8140/2   Adenocarcinoma in situ
M8140/3   Adenocarcinoma NOS
M8140/6   Adenocarcinoma, metastatic NOS
M8141/3   Scirrhous adenocarcinoma
M8146/0   Monomorphic adenoma
M8147/0   Basal cell adenoma
M8190/0   Trabecular adenoma
M8190/3   Trabecular adenocarcinoma
M8200/3   Adenoid cystic carcinoma NOS
              Cylindroma NOS
              Adenocarcinoma, cylindroid type
M8201/3   Cribriform carcinoma
M8211/0   Tubular adenoma NOS
M8211/3   Tubular adenocarcinoma
M8230/3   Solid carcinoma NOS
M8250/3   Bronchiolo-alveolar adenocarcinoma
M8251/0   Alveolar adenoma
M8260/0   Papillary adenoma NOS
M8260/3   Papillary adenocarcinoma NOS
M8290/0   Oxyphilic adenoma
              Oncocytic adenoma
              Oncocytoma
M8290/3   Oxyphilic adenocarcinoma
              Oncocytic carcinoma
              Oncocytic adenocarcinoma
M8300/0   Basophil adenoma
M8300/3   Basophil carcinoma
M8310/0   Clear cell adenoma
M8310/3   Clear cell adenocarcinoma NOS
M8312/3   Renal cell carcinoma
              Renal cell adenocarcinoma
              Grawitz' tumour
              Hypernephroma
M8320/3   Granular cell carcinoma
M8340/3   Papillary carcinoma, follicular variant
              Papillary and follicular adenocarcinoma

M843   Mucoepidermoid neoplasms
M8430/1   Mucoepidermoid tumour
M8430/3   Mucoepidermoid carcinoma

135

M844–M849   Cystic, mucinous and serous neoplasms
M8440/0   Cystadenoma NOS
M8440/3   Cystadenocarcinoma NOS
M8450/0   Papillary cystadenoma NOS
M8450/3   Papillary cystadenocarcinoma NOS

M850–M854   Ductal, lobular and medullary neoplasms
M8510/3   Medullary carcinoma NOS
          Medullary adenocarcinoma

M855   Acinar cell neoplasms
M8550/0   Acinar cell adenoma
          Acinar adenoma
          Acinic cell adenoma
M8550/1   Acinar cell tumour
          Acinic cell tumour
M8550/3   Acinar cell carcinoma
          Acinic cell adenocarcinoma
          Acinar adenocarcinoma
          Acinar carcinoma

M856–M858   Complex epithelial neoplasms
M8560/3   Adenosquamous carcinoma
          Mixed adenocarcinoma and squamous cell carcinoma
          Mixed adenocarcinoma and epidermoid carcinoma
M8561/0   Adenolymphoma
          Papillary cystadenoma lymphomatosum
          Warthin's tumour
M8562/3   Epithelial-myoepithelial carcinoma
M8570/3   Adenocarcinoma with squamous metaplasia
M8571/3   Adenocarcinoma with cartilaginous and osseous metaplasia
          Adenocarcinoma with cartilaginous metaplasia
          Adenocarcinoma with osseous metaplasia

M868–M871   Paragangliomas and glomus tumours
M8692/1   Carotid body tumour
          Carotid body paraganglioma
M8700/0   Phaeochromocytoma NOS
M8700/3   Phaeochromocytoma, malignant
M8711/0   Glomus tumour
M8712/0   Glomangioma

M872–M879   Naevi and melanomas
M8720/0   Pigmented naevus NOS
M8720/2   Melanoma in situ

M8720/3   Malignant melanoma NOS
M8722/3   Balloon cell melanoma
M8730/0   Nonpigmented naevus
M8730/3   Amelanotic melanoma
M8740/0   Junctional naevus
          Junction naevus
          Intraepidermal naevus
M8740/3   Malignant melanoma in junctional naevus
M8741/2   Precancerous melanosis NOS
M8741/3   Malignant melanoma in precancerous melanosis
M8742/2   Hutchinson's melanotic freckle
          Lentigo maligna
M8742/3   Malignant melanoma in Hutchinson's melanotic freckle
M8743/3   Superficial spreading melanoma
M8750/0   Intradermal naevus
          Dermal naevus
M8760/0   Compound naevus
M8770/0   Epithelioid and spindle cell naevus
          Juvenile naevus
          Juvenile melanoma
M8771/0   Epithelioid cell naevus
M8772/0   Spindle cell naevus
M8772/3   Spindle cell melanoma
M8780/0   Blue naevus NOS
M8780/3   Blue naevus, malignant
M8790/0   Cellular blue naevus

M880   Soft tissue tumours and sarcomas NOS
M8800/0   Soft tissue tumour, benign
M8800/3   Sarcoma NOS
M8801/3   Spindle cell sarcoma
M8802/3   Giant cell sarcoma (except of bone M9250/3)
          Pleomorphic cell sarcoma

M881–M883   Fibromatous neoplasms
M8810/0   Fibroma NOS
M8810/3   Fibrosarcoma NOS
M8811/0   Fibromyxoma (myxoma of jaw M9320/0)
M8811/3   Fibromyxosarcoma
M8812/3   Periosteal fibrosarcoma
M8821/1   Aggressive fibromatosis
          Extra-abdominal desmoid
          Desmoid NOS
          Invasive fibroma

137

M8823/1   Desmoplastic fibroma
M8830/0   Fibrous histiocytoma NOS
          Fibroxanthoma
M8830/3   Fibrous histiocytoma, malignant
M8832/0   Dermatofibroma NOS

M884   Myxomatous neoplasms
M8840/0   Myxoma NOS (Myxoma of jaw M9320/0)
M8840/3   Myxosarcoma

M885–M888   Lipomatous neoplasms
M8850/0   Lipoma NOS
M8850/3   Liposarcoma NOS
M8851/0   Fibrolipoma
          Fibroma molle

M889–M892   Myomatous neoplasms
M8890/0   Leiomyoma NOS
          Fibromyoma
          Leiomyofibroma
          Myofibroma
M8890/3   Leiomyosarcoma NOS
M8894/0   Angiomyoma
          Vascular leiomyoma
M8900/0   Rhabdomyoma
M8900/3   Rhabdomyosarcoma NOS
M8910/3   Embryonal rhabdomyosarcoma
M8920/3   Alveolar rhabdomyosarcoma

M893–M899   Complex mixed and stromal neoplasms
M8940/0   Pleomorphic adenoma
          Mixed tumour NOS
          Mixed tumour, salivary gland type NOS
M8940/3   Mixed tumour, malignant
M8941/3   Carcinoma in pleomorphic adenoma
M8980/3   Carcinosarcoma NOS
M8982/0   Myoepithelioma
M8990/3   Mesenchymoma, malignant

M904   Synovial-like neoplasms
M9040/0   Synovioma, benign
M9040/3   Synovial sarcoma NOS

M906–M909 Germ cell neoplasms
M9080/0   Teratoma, benign
M9080/1   Teratoma NOS
M9080/3   Teratoma, malignant NOS
M9084/0   Dermoid cyst NOS

M912–M916 Blood vessel tumours
M9120/0   Haemangioma NOS
M9120/3   Haemangiosarcoma
M9121/0   Cavernous haemangioma
M9130/0   Haemangioendothelioma, benign
M9130/1   Haemangioendothelioma NOS
M9130/3   Haemangioendothelioma, malignant
M9131/0   Capillary haemangioma
M9140/3   Kaposi's sarcoma
M9150/0   Haemangiopericytoma, benign
M9150/1   Haemangiopericytoma NOS
M9150/3   Haemangiopericytoma, malignant
M9160/0   Angiofibroma NOS

M917 Lymphatic vessel tumours
M9170/0   Lymphangioma NOS
M9170/3   Lymphangiosarcoma
M9171/0   Capillary lymphangioma
M9172/0   Cavernous lymphangioma
M9173/0   Cystic lymphangioma
               Cystic hygroma
M9175/0   Haemolymphangioma

M918–M924 Osseous and chondromatous neoplasms
M9180/0   Osteoma NOS
M9180/3   Osteosarcoma NOS
M9181/3   Chondroblastic osteosarcoma
M9182/3   Fibroblastic osteosarcoma
M9183/3   Telangiectatic osteosarcoma
M9184/3   Osteosarcoma in Paget's disease of bone
M9190/3   Juxtacortical osteosarcoma
               Parosteal osteosarcoma
               Periosteal osteogenic sarcoma
M9191/0   Osteoid osteoma NOS
M9200/0   Osteoblastoma
M9210/0   Osteochondroma
M9220/0   Chondroma NOS
M9220/3   Chondrosarcoma NOS

M9221/0   Juxtacortical chondroma
M9221/3   Juxtacortical chondrosarcoma
M9240/3   Mesenchymal chondrosarcoma
M9241/0   Chondromyxoid fibroma

M925   Giant cell tumours
M9250/1   Giant cell tumour of bone NOS
M9250/3   Giant cell tumour of bone, malignant

M926   Miscellaneous bone tumours
M9260/3   Ewing's sarcoma
M9262/0   Ossifying fibroma[1]
          Fibro-osteoma
          Osteofibroma

M927–M934 Odontogenic tumours[1]
M9270/0   Odontogenic tumour, benign
M9270/1   Odontogenic tumour NOS
M9270/3   Odontogenic tumour, malignant
          Odontogenic carcinoma
          Odontogenic sarcoma
          Intraosseous carcinoma
          Ameloblastic carcinoma
M9271/0   Dentinoma
M9272/0   Cementoma NOS
M9273/0   Cementoblastoma, benign
M9274/0   Cementifying fibroma
M9275/0   Gigantiform cementoma
          Florid (cemento-)osseous dysplasia
M9280/0   Odontoma NOS
M9281/0   Compound odontoma
M9282/0   Complex odontoma
M9290/0   Ameloblastic fibro-odontoma
          Fibroameloblastic odontoma
M9290/3   Ameloblastic odontosarcoma
M9300/0   Adenomatoid odontogenic tumour
          Adenoameloblastoma
M9301/0   Calcifying odontogenic cyst
M9302/0   Odontogenic ghost cell tumour

---

[1] See also Annex 1, Histological typing of odontogenic tumours, which contains significant differences.

M9310/0	Ameloblastoma NOS
	Adamantinoma NOS
M9310/3	Ameloblastoma, malignant
	Adamantinoma, malignant
M9311/0	Odontoameloblastoma
M9312/0	Squamous odontogenic tumour
M9320/0	Odontogenic myxoma
	Odontogenic myxofibroma
M9321/0	Central odontogenic fibroma
M9322/0	Peripheral odontogenic fibroma
M9330/0	Ameloblastic fibroma
M9330/3	Ameloblastic fibrosarcoma
	Ameloblastic sarcoma
	Odontogenic fibrosarcoma
M9340/0	Calcifying epithelial odontogenic tumour
	Pindborg tumour

M935–M937   Miscellaneous tumours

M9350/1	Craniopharyngioma
M9363/0	Melanotic neuroectodermal tumour
M9370/3	Chordoma

M949–M952   Neuroepitheliomatous neoplasms

| M9500/3 | Neuroblastoma NOS |
| M9510/3 | Retinoblastoma NOS |

M953   Meningiomas

| M9530/0 | Meningioma NOS |

M954–M957   Nerve sheath tumours

M9540/0	Neurofibroma NOS
M9540/1	Neurofibromatosis NOS
M9540/3	Neurofibrosarcoma
M9541/0	Melanotic neurofibroma
M9550/0	Plexiform neurofibroma
M9560/0	Neurilemmoma NOS
M9560/3	Neurilemmoma, malignant
M9570/0	Neuroma NOS

M958   Granular cell tumours and alveolar soft part sarcoma

M9580/0	Granular cell tumour NOS
	Granular cell myoblastoma NOS
M9580/3	Granular cell tumour, malignant
M9581/3	Alveolar soft part sarcoma

M959–M970   Hodgkin's and non-Hodgkin's lymphoma

M959   Malignant lymphomas NOS or diffuse
M9590/3   Malignant lymphoma NOS
M9591/3   Malignant lymphoma, non-Hodgkin's NOS
M9592/3   Lymphosarcoma NOS
M9593/3   Reticulosarcoma NOS

M965–M966   Hodgkin's disease
M9650/3   Hodgkin's disease NOS
M9661/3   Hodgkin's granuloma

M967–M968   Malignant lymphoma, diffuse or NOS, specified type
M9687/3   Burkitt's lymphoma NOS

M969   Malignant lymphoma, follicular or nodular, with or without diffuse areas

M970   Specified cutaneous and peripheral T-cell lymphomas
M9700/3   Mycosis fungoides

M972   Other lymphoreticular neoplasms
M9720/3   Malignant histiocytosis
M9722/3   Letterer–Siwe disease

M973   Plasma cell tumours
M9731/3   Plasmacytoma NOS
M9732/3   Multiple myeloma
Myelomatosis

M976   Immunoproliferative diseases
M9761/3   Waldenström's macroglobulinaemia

M980–M994   Leukaemias

M980   Leukaemias NOS
M9800/3   Leukaemia NOS
M9801/3   Acute leukaemia NOS
M9803/3   Chronic leukaemia NOS
M9804/3   Aleukaemic leukaemia NOS

M982   Lymphoid leukaemias
M9820/3   Lymphoid leukaemia NOS

M984   Erythroleukaemias
M9841/3   Acute erythraemia

M986   Myeloid (granulocytic) leukaemias
M9860/3   Myeloid leukaemia NOS

M989   Monocytic leukaemias
M9890/3   Monocytic leukaemia NOS

M990–M994   Other leukaemias
M9930/3   Myeloid sarcoma

M995–M997   Miscellaneous myeloproliferative and lymphoproliferative disorders
M9950/1   Polycythaemia vera

Annex 1

Histological typing of odontogenic tumours[1]

1. Neoplasms and other tumours related to the odontogenic apparatus

1.1	Benign	
1.1.1	Odontogenic epithelium without odontogenic ectomesenchyme	
1.1.1.1	Ameloblastoma	9310/0[2]
1.1.1.2	Squamous odontogenic tumour	9312/0
1.1.1.3	Calcifying epithelial odontogenic tumour (Pindborg tumour)	9340/0
1.1.1.4	Clear cell odontogenic tumour	9270/0
1.1.2	Odontogenic epithelium with odontogenic ectomesenchyme, with or without dental hard tissue formation	
1.1.2.1	Ameloblastic fibroma	9330/0
1.1.2.2	Ameloblastic fibrodentinoma (dentinoma) and ameloblastic fibro-odontoma	9290/0
1.1.2.3	Odontoameloblastoma	9311/0
1.1.2.4	Adenomatoid odontogenic tumour	9300/0
1.1.2.5	Calcifying odontogenic cyst	9301/0
1.1.2.6	Complex odontoma	9282/0
1.1.2.7	Compound odontoma	9281/0
1.1.3	Odontogenic ectomesenchyme with or without included odontogenic epithelium	
1.1.3.1	Odontogenic fibroma	See note 1
1.1.3.2	Myxoma (odontogenic myxoma, myxofibroma)	9320/0
1.1.3.3	Benign cementoblastoma (cementoblastoma, true cementoma)	9273/0

---

[1] Extracted from: Kramer IRH, Pindborg JJ, Shear M. *Histological typing of odontogenic tumours*, 2nd ed. Berlin, Springer-Verlag, 1992.
[2] Morphology code of the International Classification of Diseases for Oncology (ICD-O) and the Systematized Nomenclature of Medicine (SNOMED).

1.2   Malignant

1.2.1   Odontogenic carcinomas
1.2.1.1   Malignant ameloblastoma 9310/3
1.2.1.2   Primary intraosseous carcinoma. 9270/3
1.2.1.3   Malignant variants of other odontogenic epithelial
           tumours. . . . . .See note 2
1.2.1.4   Malignant changes in odontogenic cysts 9270/3
1.2.2   Odontogenic sarcomas
1.2.2.1   Ameloblastic fibrosarcoma (ameloblastic sarcoma) 9330/3
1.2.2.2   Ameloblastic fibrodentinosarcoma and ameloblastic
           fibro-odontosarcoma 9290/3
1.2.3   Odontogenic carcinosarcoma 8980/3

2. Neoplasms and other tumours related to bone

2.1   Osteogenic neoplasms

2.1.1   Cemento-ossifying fibroma (cementifying fibroma,
           ossifying fibroma) . . . . .See note 3

2.2   Non-neoplastic bone lesions

2.2.1   Fibrous dysplasia of the jaws 74910
2.2.2   Cemento-osseous dysplasia
2.2.2.1   Periapical cemental dysplasia (periapical fibrous
           dysplasia) 9272/0
2.2.2.2   Florid cemento-osseous dysplasia (gigantiform
           cementoma, familial multiple cementomas) 9275/0
2.2.2.3   Other cemento-osseous dysplasias
2.2.3   Cherubism (familial multilocular cystic disease of the
           jaws). 70980
2.2.4   Central giant cell granuloma 44130
2.2.5   Aneurysmal bone cyst 33640
2.2.6   Solitary bone cyst (traumatic, simple, haemorrhagic
           bone cyst). 33404

2.3   Other tumours

2.3.1   Melanotic neuroectodermal tumour of infancy
           (melanotic progonoma). 9363/0

3. Epithelial cysts

3.1   Developmental

3.1.1   Odontogenic
3.1.1.1   "Gingival cyst" of infants (Epstein pearls) 26540
3.1.1.2   Odontogenic keratocyst (primordial cyst) 26530
3.1.1.3   Dentigerous (follicular) cyst 26560
3.1.1.4   Eruption cyst 26550
3.1.1.5   Lateral periodontal cyst 26520
3.1.1.6   Gingival cyst of adults 26540
3.1.1.7   Glandular odontogenic cyst; sialo-odontogenic cyst 26520
3.1.2   Nonodontogenic
3.1.2.1   Nasopalatine duct (incisive canal) cyst 26600
3.1.2.2   Nasolabial (nasoalveolar) cyst 26500

3.2   Inflammatory

3.2.1   Radicular cyst 43800
3.2.1.1   Apical and lateral radicular cyst
3.2.1.2   Residual radicular cyst
3.3.2   Paradental (inflammatory collateral, mandibular
            infected buccal) cyst 26520

Note 1: Central odontogenic fibroma 9321/0, peripheral odontogenic fibroma
           9322/0.
Note 2: Use appropriate tumour coding from 1.1 above, with behaviour
           code /3.
Note 3: Ossifying fibroma 9262/0, cementifying fibroma 9274/0.
           9262/0 is recommended for cemento-ossifying fibroma.

Annex 2

Histological typing of salivary gland tumours[1]

1. Adenomas

1.1	Pleomorphic adenoma	.8940/0[2]
1.2	Myoepithelioma (myoepithelial adenoma)	.8982/0
1.3	Basal cell adenoma	.8147/0
1.4	Warthin tumour (adenolymphoma)	.8561/0
1.5	Oncocytoma (Oncocytic adenoma)	.8290/0
1.6	Canalicular adenoma	
1.7	Sebaceous adenoma	.8410/0
1.8	Ductal papilloma	.8503/0
1.8.1	Inverted ductal papilloma	.8053/0
1.8.2	Intraductal papilloma	.8503/0
1.8.3	Sialadenoma papilliferum	.8260/0
1.9	Cystadenoma	.8440/0
1.9.1	Papillary cystadenoma	.8450/0
1.9.2	Mucinous cystadenoma	.8470/0

2. Carcinomas

2.1	Acinic cell carcinoma	.8550/3
2.2	Mucoepidermoid carcinoma	.8430/3
2.3	Adenoid cystic carcinoma	.8200/3
2.4	Polymorphous low grade adenocarcinoma (terminal duct adenocarcinoma)	
2.5	Epithelial-myoepithelial carcinoma	.8562/3
2.6	Basal cell adenocarcinoma	.8147/3
2.7	Sebaceous carcinoma	.8410/3
2.8	Papillary cystadenocarcinoma	.8450/3
2.9	Mucinous adenocarcinoma	.8480/3
2.10	Oncocytic carcinoma	.8290/3

---

[1] Extracted from: Seifert G. *Histological typing of salivary gland tumours*, 2nd ed. Berlin, Springer-Verlag, 1991.
[2] Morphology code of the International Classification of Diseases for Oncology (ICD-O) and the Systematized Nomenclature of Medicine (SNOMED).

3. Non-epithelial tumours

4. Malignant lymphomas

5. Secondary tumours

6. Unclassified tumours

7. Tumour-like lesions

Index

Abrasion of teeth K03.1
– dentifrice K03.10
– habitual K03.11
– occupational K03.12
– ritual K03.13
– traditional K03.13

Abscess (of)
– cutaneous
– – face L02.0
– – neck L02.1
– dental
– – without sinus K04.7
– – with sinus K04.6
– lymph node, acute L04.–
– mouth K12.2X
– periapical (dentoalveolar)
– – without sinus K04.7
– – with sinus (to) K04.6
– – – maxillary antrum K04.60
– – – nasal cavity K04.61
– – – NOS K04.69
– – – oral cavity K04.62
– – – skin K04.63
– periodontal [parodontal]
– – gingival origin
– – – without sinus K05.20
– – – with sinus K05.21
– – pulpal origin
– – – without sinus K04.7
– – – with sinus K04.6
– peritonsillar J36
– phaeomycotic B43.–
– postprocedural T81.4
– pulpal K04.02

Abscess (of) (*continued*)
– salivary gland K11.3
– stitch T81.4
– submandibular K12.2X
– tongue K14.00
– wound T81.4

Acanthosis nigricans L83.XX

Acatalasia E80.3X

Accretions (*see* **Deposits on teeth**)

Achondroplasia Q77.4X

Acrocephalosyndactyly Q87.00

Acrocephaly Q75.00

Acrodermatitis
– continua L40.2X
– enteropathica E83.2X

Acrodynia T56.1

Acrokeratosis verruciformis Q82.85

Actinomycosis, cervicofacial A42.2X

Adamantinoma
– malignant M9310/3
– NOS M9310/0

Addison's disease E27.1X

Adenoameloblastoma M9300/0

Adenocarcinoma
– acinar M8550/3
– acinic cell M8550/3
– bronchiolo-alveolar M8250/3
– clear cell NOS M8310/3
– cylindroid type M8200/3
– in situ M8140/2
– medullary M8510/3

- metastatic NOS M8140/6
- NOS M8140/3
- oncocytic M8290/3
- oxyphilic M8290/3
- papillary
- – and follicular M8340/3
- – NOS M8260/3
- renal cell M8312/3
- scirrhous M8141/3
- trabecular M8190/3
- tubular M8211/3
- with cartilaginous and osseous metaplasia M8571/3
- with cartilaginous metaplasia M8571/3
- with osseous metaplasia M8571/3
- with squamous metaplasia M8570/3

Adenolymphoma M8561/0

Adenoma
- acinar M8550/0
- acinar cell M8550/0
- acinic cell M8550/0
- alveolar M8251/0
- basal cell M8147/0
- basophil M8300/0
- clear cell M8310/0
- monomorphic M8146/0
- NOS M8140/0
- oncocytic M8290/0
- oxyphilic M8290/0
- papillary NOS M8260/0
- pleomorphic M8940/0
- trabecular M8190/0
- tubular NOS M8211/0

Adrenal gland disorder NEC E27.–

Adrenocortical insufficiency, primary E27.1

Adverse effects (*see* individual drugs and drug types)

Adverse incidents, associated with
- miscellaneous devices, NEC Y82.8

Adverse incidents, associated with (*continued*)
- prosthetic devices and other implants Y82.2
- surgical instruments and devices Y82.3

Aerodontalgia T70.2

Aerosol propellants, toxic effect T59

Agammaglobulinaemia D80.VX

Aglossia Q38.30

Agranulocytosis D70.–

AIDS NOS B24.XX

AIDS-related complex B24.XX

Air pressure, effects of T70.–

Albers–Schönberg syndrome Q78.2X

Albright(–McCune)(–Sternberg) syndrome Q78.1

Alcohol, toxic effect T51

Allergy NOS T78.4

Altitude, effects of, NEC T70.2

Alveolitis of jaw K10.3

Alveolus, alveolar
- fracture S02.8
- process
- – irregular K08.81
- – mandibular, fracture S02.60
- – maxillary, fracture S02.40
- ridge
- – atrophy K08.2X
- – carcinoma in situ D00.02
- – enlargement NOS K08.82
- – neoplasm
- – – benign D10.33
- – – malignant C03.–

Ameloblastoma
– malignant M9310/3
– NOS M9310/0

Amelogenesis imperfecta K00.50

Amyloidosis E85.VX

Anaemia
– aplastic D61.VX
– Cooley's D56.VX
– deficiency
– – folate D52.VX
– – iron D50.–
– – – secondary to blood loss D50.0X
– – vitamin B_{12} D51.VX
– due to enzyme disorder D55.VX
– haemolytic
– – acquired D59.VX
– – hereditary D58.VX
– Mediterranean D56.VX
– nutritional D53.VX
– sickle-cell D57.VX

Anaesthesia of skin R20.0

Anaesthetics
– inhaled, adverse effects Y48.0X
– local, adverse effects Y48.3X
– poisoning T41

Analgesics
– adverse effects Y45.–
– nonopioid, poisoning T39

Aneurysm, arteriovenous, of mandible Q27.3X

Angina
– agranulocytic D70.X0
– Vincent's A69.11

Angiofibroma NOS M9160/0

Angiomyoma M8894/0

Angioneurotic oedema T78.3

Ankyloglossia Q38.1

Ankylosis of teeth K03.5

Anodontia K00.0
– partial K00.00
– total K00.01

Anomalies
– dentofacial (of) K07.–
– – dental arch K07.2
– – functional K07.5
– – jaw–cranial base relationship K07.1
– – jaw size, major K07.0
– of tooth position

Anorexia nervosa F50.VX

Anthrax A22.8X

Antibiotics
– local, poisoning T49.0
– systemic
– – adverse effects Y40.–
– – poisoning T36

Antiepileptic drugs
– adverse effects Y46.–
– poisoning T42

Antifungal drugs NEC
– local
– – adverse effects Y56.0X
– – poisoning T49.0
– systemic, adverse effects Y40.7X

Anti-infectives NEC
– local
– – adverse effects Y56.0X
– – poisoning T49.0
– systemic
– – adverse effects Y41.9X
– – poisoning T37

Anti-inflammatory drugs
– adverse effects Y45.–
– local, NEC
– – adverse effects Y56.0X
– – poisoning T49.0
– nonsteroidal, adverse effects Y45.3X

Antimalarials, adverse effects Y41.2X

Antineoplastic drugs NEC, adverse effects Y43.3X

Antiparasitics NEC
– adverse effects Y41.9X
– poisoning T37

Antiparkinsonism drugs
– adverse effects Y46.–
– poisoning T42

Antipyretics
– adverse effects Y45.–
– poisoning T39

Antirheumatics
– adverse effects Y45.4X
– poisoning T39

Antiviral drugs, adverse effects Y41.5X

Aorta, coarctation Q25.1X

Apert's syndrome Q87.00

Aphasia R47.0

Aphthae
– Bednar's K12.03
– major K12.01
– Mikulicz' K12.00
– minor K12.00
– oral K12.0
– recurrent K12.0
– Sutton's K12.01

Aplasia, cementum K00.43

Arsenic, toxic effect T57.0

Arteries, congenital malformations Q25.–

Arteriovenous
– aneurysm of mandible Q27.3X
– malformation, peripheral Q27.3X

Arteritis, giant cell, NEC M31.6X

Arthritis, temporomandibular joint
– juvenile M08.VX
– NOS M13.9X
– pyogenic M00.VX
– rheumatoid M06.VX
– – seropositive M05.VX

Arthropathy, temporomandibular joint
– reactive M02.3X
– traumatic M12.5X

Arthropod-borne viral fever A93.8

Arthrosis, temporomandibular joint M19.0X

Ascariasis B77.VX

Ascorbic acid deficiency E54.XX

Aspergillosis B44.8X

Astringents, local, poisoning T49.2

Asymmetry
– jaw K07.10
– facial Q67.0

Atresia of salivary gland or duct Q38.42

Atrophy
– edentulous alveolar ridge K08.2X
– hemifacial Q76.41
– salivary glands K11.0
– tongue papillae K14.4
– – due to cleaning habits K14.40
– – due to systemic disorder K14.41

Attrition of teeth, excessive K03.0
– approximal K03.01
– occlusal K03.00

Avulsion of tooth S03.22

Behçet's disease M35.2X

Bejel A65.XX

Bell's palsy G51.0

Beriberi E51.1X

Biting, cheek and lip K13.1

Black eye S00.1

Blastomycosis B40.VX
– Brazilian B41.VX

Blockers, calcium-channel, adverse effects Y52.1X

Blushing, excessive R23.2

Bourneville's disease Q85.1X

Bowen's disease M8081/2

Branchial cleft sinus, fistula and cyst Q18.0

Brazilian blastomycosis B41.VX

Breathing, mouth R06.5

Brucella melitensis, **brucellosis A23.0X**

Bruxism F45.82

Bulimia F50.VX

Bullous disease of childhood, chronic L12.2X

Burkitt's tumour M9687/3, C83.7X
– – due to HIV disease B21.1X

Burn
– head and neck T20.–
– – first degree T20.1
– – second degree T20.2
– – sequelae T95.0
– – third degree T20.3
– mouth and pharynx T28.0

Café au lait spots L81.3X

Calcification of muscle M61.VX

Calcium
– deficiency, dietary E58.XX
– metabolism, disorder E83.5X

Calcium-channel blockers, adverse effects Y52.1X

Calculus
– in duct K11.5X
– subgingival K03.65
– supragingival K03.64

Cancrum oris A69.0

Candidiasis, candidosis B37.–
– due to HIV disease B20.4X
– mucocutaneous B37.04

Canker sore K12.00

Carbohydrate metabolism disorder E74.–

Carbon monoxide, toxic effect T58

Carbuncle
– face L02.0
– neck L02.1

Carcinoma
– acinar M8550/3
– acinar cell M8550/3
– adenoid cystic NOS M8200/3

– adenosquamous M8560/3
– ameloblastic M9270/3
– anaplastic NOS M8021/3
– basal cell NOS M8090/3
– – multicentric M8091/3
– basophil M8300/3
– basosquamous M8094/3
– cribriform M8201/3
– epidermoid NOS M8070/3
– epithelial-myoepithelial M8562/3
– granular cell M8320/3
– in pleomorphic adenoma M8941/3
– in situ
– – alveolar ridge D00.02
– – epidermoid
– – – NOS M8070/2
– – – with questionable stromal invasion M8076/2
– – gingiva D00.02
– – lip
– – – skin D04.0
– – – vermilion border D00.00
– – mouth, floor D00.04
– – mucosa
– – – buccal D00.01
– – – labial D00.00
– – nasal cavity D02.3X
– – NOS M8010/2
– – oropharynx D00.07
– – palate D00.03
– – sinus, accessory D02.3X
– – skin
– – – face D04.3
– – – lip D04.0
– – squamous cell
– – – NOS M8070/2
– – – with questionable stromal invasion M8076/2
– – tongue D00.06
– – – ventral surface D00.05
– intraepidermal NOS M8070/2
– intraepithelial NOS M8010/2
– intraosseous M9270/3
– lymphoepithelial M8082/3
– medullary NOS M8510/3
– mucoepidermoid M8430/3

Carcinoma (*continued*)
- NOS M8010/3
- - metastatic M8010/6
- oat cell M8042/3
- odontogenic M9270/3
- oncocytic M8290/3
- papillary
- - follicular variant M8340/3
- - NOS M8050/3
- pleomorphic M8022/3
- pseudosarcomatous M8033/3
- renal cell M8312/3
- round cell M8041/3
- secondary M8010/6
- small cell NOS M8041/3
- solid M8230/3
- squamous M8070/3
- squamous cell
- - adenoid type M8075/3
- - intraepidermal, Bowen's type M8081/2
- - intraepithelial M8070/2
- - keratinizing NOS M8071/3
- - metastatic NOS M8070/6
- - microinvasive M8076/3
- - NOS M8070/3
- - papillary M8052/3
- - spindle cell M8074/3
- transitional cell, spindle cell type M8122/3
- undifferentiated NOS M8020/3
- verrucous M8051/3

Carcinosarcoma NOS M8980/3

Cardiac septa, congenital malformations Q21.–

Caries K02.–
- arrested K02.3
- cementum K02.2
- dentine K02.1
- enamel K02.1
- initial K02.1

Cat-scratch disease A28.10

Catalase defects E80.3

Cellulitis
– face L03.2
– head and neck L03.8X
– mouth K12.2X

Cementoblastoma, benign M9273/0

Cementoma
– gigantiform M9275/0
– NOS M9272/0

Cervical fusion syndrome Q76.1

Chagas' disease B57.VX

Cheek
– biting K13.1
– internal, superficial injury S00.50
– open wound S01.4

Cheilitis
– actinic L57.0X
– angular K13.00
– – candidal B37.06
– exfoliative K13.02
– glandularis apostematosa K13.01
– NOS K13.03

Cheilodynia K13.04

Cheilosis, angular K13.00

Cherubism K10.80

Chickenpox B01.8X

Chloramphenicol group antibiotics, adverse effects Y40.2X

Chondroma
– juxtacortical M9221/0
– NOS M9220/0

Chondrosarcoma
– juxtacortical M9221/3

Chondrosarcoma (*continued*)
– mesenchymal M9240/3
– NOS M9220/3

Chordoma M9370/3

Chromomycosis B43.8X

Chromosome
– abnormalities
– – deletion of short arm
– – – chromosome 4 Q93.3X
– – – chromosome 5 Q93.4X
– – NEC Q99.–
– – sex chromosomes, male phenotype Q98.–
– fragile X Q99.2X

Cleft
– lip Q36.–
– – bilateral Q36.0
– – – with cleft palate Q37.8
– – – – hard Q37.0
– – – – – and soft Q37.4
– – – – soft Q37.2
– – medial Q36.1
– – unilateral Q36.9
– – – with cleft palate NOS Q37.9
– – – – hard Q37.1
– – – – – and soft Q37.5
– – – – soft Q37.3
– – with cleft palate Q37.–
– palate Q35.–
– – hard
– – – bilateral Q35.0
– – – unilateral Q35.1
– – – with cleft lip
– – – – bilateral Q37.0
– – – – unilateral Q37.1
– – hard and soft
– – – bilateral Q35.4
– – – unilateral Q35.5
– – – with cleft lip
– – – – bilateral Q37.4
– – – – unilateral Q37.5
– – medial Q35.6

- – soft
- – – bilateral Q35.2
- – – unilateral Q35.3
- – – with cleft lip
- – – – bilateral Q37.2
- – – – unilateral Q37.3
- – uvula Q35.7

Clotting factor deficiency, hereditary D68.2X

Coagulation
- defects D68.–
- disseminated intravascular D65.XX
- factor deficiency, acquired D68.4X

Coarctation of aorta Q25.1X

Cocaine, self-poisoning X62.VX

Coccidioidomycosis B38.VX

Colour change
- dental hard tissue, posteruptive, due to
- – chewing habit
- – – betel K03.72
- – – tobacco K03.72
- – metals, metallic compounds K03.70
- – pulpal bleeding K03.71
- tooth, during formation, due to
- – biliary system malformation K00.81
- – blood type incompatibility K00.80
- – porphyria K00.82
- – tetracyclines K00.83

Complications (of)
- infusion procedure T80
- injection, therapeutic T80
- mechanical, due to
- – bone graft T84.3
- – bone stimulator, electronic T84.3
- – internal fixation of bones T84.2
- – joint prosthesis T84.0
- – muscle graft T84.4

Complications (of) (*continued*)
– mechanical, due to (*continued*)
– – tendon graft T84.4
– procedure NEC T81.–
– transfusion procedure T80

Compression facies Q67.1

Concrescence K00.22

Condition
– Fordyce Q38.60
– haemorrhagic NOS D69.9X
– inflammatory, of jaws K10.2

Condyloma acuminatum, oral B07.X1

Contact dermatitis
– allergic, due to cosmetics L23.2X
– irritant L24.VX

Contraceptives, oral, adverse effects Y42.4X

Cooley's anaemia D56.VX

Corrosion
– head and neck T20.–
– – first degree T20.4
– – second degree T20.5
– – sequelae T95.0
– – third degree T20.7
– mouth and pharynx T28.5

Corrosive substances, toxic effect T54

Costen's syndrome K07.60

Cranial nerves, injury S04.–

Craniopharyngioma M9350/1

Craniosynostosis Q75.0

Cri-du-chat syndrome Q93.4X

Crohn's disease K50.8X

Crossbite (anterior) (posterior) K07.25

Crowding, teeth K07.30

Cryptococcosis B45.8X

Cyanosis R23.0X

Cylindroma NOS M8200/3

Cyst (of)
- apical periodontal K04.8
- branchial cleft Q18.0
- – site of neoplasm C10.4
- calcifying odontogenic M9301/0
- dentigerous K09.03
- dermoid M9084/0, K09.80
- developmental
- – nonodontogenic K09.1
- – odontogenic K09.0
- epidermoid K09.81
- eruption K09.00
- follicular K09.03
- gingival
- – developmental K09.01
- – of adult K06.80
- – of newborn K09.82
- globulomaxillary K09.10
- incisive canal K09.12
- jaw K09.2
- – aneurysmal bone K09.20
- – epithelial K09.22
- – haemorrhagic K09.21
- – latent K10.02
- – solitary bone K09.21
- – static K10.02
- – traumatic K09.21
- lateral periodontal K09.04
- lymphoepithelial K09.85
- maxillary sinus J34.1X
- median palatal K09.11
- mucous extravasation K11.61
- mucous retention K11.60
- nasoalveolar K09.84

Cyst (of) (*continued*)
- nasolabial K09.84
- nasopalatine K09.12
- oral region, NEC K09.–
- palatal, of newborn K09.83
- palatine papilla K09.13
- periapical K04.8
- primordial K09.02
- radicular K04.8
- – apical K04.80
- – inflammatory paradental K04.82
- – lateral K04.80
- – residual K04.81
- Stafne's K10.02
- thyroglossal Q89.21

Cystadenocarcinoma
- NOS M8440/3
- papillary NOS M8450/3

Cystadenoma
- NOS M8440/0
- papillary NOS M8450/0
- – lymphomatosum M8561/0

Cystic fibrosis E84.VX

Cysticercosis B69.8X

Cytomegaloviral disease B25.8X
- due to HIV disease B20.2X

Darier–White disease Q82.81

Decompression sickness T70.3

Defect
- coagulation D68.–
- developmental bone, in mandible K10.02
- platelet, qualitative D69.1X
- septal
- – atrial Q21.1X
- – ventricular Q21.0X
- wedge K03.10

Defibrination syndrome D65.XX

Deficiency
- ascorbic acid E54.XX
- calcium, dietary E58.XX
- clotting factor, hereditary, NEC D68.2X
- coagulation factor, acquired D68.4X
- factor VIII D66.XX
- factor IX D67.XX
- factor XI D68.1X
- growth hormone, idiopathic E23.01
- niacin E52.XX
- nutrient element NEC E61.VX
- riboflavin E53.0X
- thiamine E51.–
- vitamin E56.–
- – A E50.8X
- – B group NEC E53.8X
- – D E55.–
- – K E56.1X
- zinc, dietary E60.XX

Degeneration, pulp K04.2

Dehiscence of operation wound, NEC T81.3

Dens
- evaginatus K00.24
- in dente K00.25
- invaginatus K00.25

Dental drugs, topical
- adverse effects Y56.7X
- poisoning T49.7

Dental root, retained K08.3X

Dentia praecox K00.62

Denticles K04.2

Dentifrice abrasion of teeth K03.10

Dentine, dentinal
- caries K02.1
- dysplasia K00.58

Dentine, dentinal (*continued*)
– irregular K04.3X
– secondary K04.3X
– sensitive K03.80

Dentinogenesis imperfecta K00.51

Dentinoma M9271/0

Denture
– hyperplasia K06.23
– sore mouth K12.12
– stomatitis K12.12
– – due to candidal infection B37.03

Deposits on teeth
– calculus
– – subgingival K03.65
– – supragingival K03.64
– due to
– – betel chewing K03.62
– – tobacco K03.61
– gross soft NEC K03.63
– pigmented film K03.60
– plaque K03.66

Dermatitis
– contact
– – allergic NEC L23.–
– – – due to cosmetics L23.2X
– – irritant L24.VX
– herpetiformis L13.0X
– perioral L71.0
– vesicular, herpesviral B00.1

Dermatofibroma NOS M8832/0

Dermatophytosis B35.–

Dermatopolymyositis M33.VX

Desmoid, extra-abdominal M8821/1

Detergents, toxic effect T55

Developmental disorder, speech and language F80.–

Deviation, midline K07.26

Diabetes mellitus NOS E14.XX

Diastema K07.33

Di George's syndrome D82.1X

Dilaceration K00.44

Diphtheria A36.VX

Disease (of)
– Addison's E27.1X
– bacterial, zoonotic A28.–
– Behçet's M35.2X
– blood, blood-forming organs D75.–
– bone, Paget's M88.–
– Bourneville's Q85.1X
– Bowen's M8081/2
– bullous, of childhood, chronic L12.2X
– caisson T70.3
– capillaries I78.–
– cat-scratch A28.10
– Chagas' B57.VX
– Crohn's K50.8X
– cytomegaloviral B25.8X
– – due to HIV disease B20.2X
– Darier–White Q82.81
– Dühring's L13.0X
– edentulous alveolar ridge K05.–
– Fabry(–Anderson) E75.20
– fifth B08.3X
– foot and mouth B08.8X
– Fordyce Q38.60
– Gaucher's E75.21
– glycogen storage E74.0
– granulomatous, chronic (childhood) D71.XX
– Hailey–Hailey Q82.80
– hand, foot and mouth B08.4X
– Hand–Schüller–Christian D76.01
– HIV (*see* Human immunodeficiency virus disease)
– Hodgkin's C81.VX
– hookworm B76.VX

Disease (of) (*continued*)
- jaws NEC K10.–
- – developmental K10.0
- joint NEC M25.–
- Letterer–Siwe M9722/3, C96.0X
- lingual tonsil K14.88
- lip NEC K13.0
- lymphoreticular tissue D76.–
- maple-syrup-urine E71.0X
- marble bone Q78.2X
- Mikulicz' K11.81
- motor neuron G12.2
- Niemann–Pick E75.22
- Ollier's Q78.4
- periodontal K05.–
- Paget's
- – facial bones M88.88
- – mandible M88.81
- – maxilla M88.80
- – skull M88.0
- Reiter's M02.3X
- Rendu–Osler–Weber I78.0X
- reticulohistiocytic system D76.–
- Simmond's E23.00
- Still's M08.VX
- tongue NEC K14.–
- Urbach–Wiethe E78.8X
- vesicular stomatitis virus A93.8X
- von Gierke's E74.0X
- von Recklinghausen's Q85.0X
- von Willebrand's D68.0X
- zoonotic bacterial A28.–

Dislocation (of)
- involving head and neck
- tooth S03.2

Disorder (of)
- adrenal gland NEC E27.–
- autonomic nervous system G90.–
- bone
- – continuity M84.–
- – density NEC M85.–
- – structure NEC M85.–
- bullous NEC L13.–

– capillaries I78.–
– connective tissue NEC L98.–
– – localized L94.–
– eating F50.–
– emotional and behavioural NEC F98.–
– endocrine NEC E34.8
– fibroblastic M72.–
– haemorrhagic, due to circulating anticoagulants D68.3X
– immune mechanism NEC D89.–
– joint NEC M25.–
– lipid storage E75.–
– menopausal N95.8X
– metabolism
– – amino-acid
– – – aromatic E70.–
– – – branched-chain E71.–
– – bilirubin E80.–
– – calcium E83.5X
– – carbohydrate NEC E74.–
– – fatty-acid E71.–
– – galactose E74.2
– – glycosaminoglycan E76.–
– – iron E83.1
– – lipoprotein NEC E78.8X
– – mineral E83.–
– – phosphorus E83.3
– – porphyrin E80.–
– – purine E79.–
– – pyrimidine E79.–
– – sphingolipid E75.–
– – zinc E83.2
– muscle NEC M62.–
– nerve
– – cranial
– – – fifth G50.–
– – – NEC G52.–
– – – ninth G52.1
– – – seventh G51.–
– – – twelfth G52.3
– – facial G51.–
– – glossopharyngeal G52.1
– – hypoglossal G52.3
– – trigeminal G50.–
– neutrophils, functional D71.XX

Disorder (of) (*continued*)
- parathyroid gland NEC E21.–
- perimenopausal N95.8X
- pigmentation NEC L81.–
- pituitary gland NEC E23.6
- polymorphonuclear neutrophil, functional D71.XX
- sickle-cell D57.VX
- skin
- – atrophic L90.–
- – granulomatous L92.–
- – hypertrophic L91.–
- – NEC L98.–
- soft tissue NEC M79.–
- somatoform F45.–
- speech and language, developmental F80.–
- speech articulation F80.0
- teeth NEC
- temporomandibular joint NEC M25.–
- thyroid NOS E07.9X
- tooth development and eruption K00.–
- veins NEC I87.8X
- white blood cells D72.–

Displacement, tooth K07.31

Disto-occlusion K07.20

Dolicocephaly Q67.2

Donovanosis A58.XX

Down's syndrome Q90.VX

Dry
- mouth NOS R68.2
- socket K10.3

Dühring's disease L13.0X

Dysautonomia, familial G90.1X

Dyskeratosis congenita Q82.83

Dyskinesia, orofacial G24.4

Dysostosis
– craniofacial Q75.1
– mandibulofacial Q75.4
– oculomandibular Q75.5

Dysphagia R13
– psychogenic F45.80
– sideropenic D50.1X

Dysphasia R47.0

Dysplasia
– chondroectodermal Q77.6X
– dentinal K00.58
– ectodermal (anhidrotic) Q82.4X
– fibrous K10.83
– florid (cemento-)osseous M9275/0
– mucoepithelial, hereditary L98.80
– polyostotic fibrous Q78.1X
– progressive diaphyseal Q78.3

Dystonia, idiopathic orofacial G24.4

Dystrophy, adiposogenital E23.60

Ear
– burn and corrosion T20.–
– open wound S01.3
– superficial injury S00.4

Eating disorder F50.–

Ecchymoses, spontaneous R23.3X

Echinococcosis B67.9X

Eczema herpeticum B00.0

Edwards' syndrome Q91.3X

Ehlers–Danlos syndrome Q79.6X

Ellis–van Creveld syndrome Q77.6X

Embedded teeth
– abnormal position K07.35
– normal position K01.0

Emphysema (subcutaneous) resulting from a procedure T81.8

En coup de sabre lesion L94.1X

Enamel
– caries K02.0
– changes due to irradiation K03.81
– hypoplasia K00.40
– – neonatal K00.42
– – prenatal K00.41
– mottling
– – endemic (fluoride) K00.30
– – non-endemic K00.31
– opacities, non-fluoride K00.31
– pearls K00.27

Enameloma K00.27

Endocrine
– disorder NEC E34.8
– glands, congenital malformations Q89.2

Enlargement (of)
– gingival K06.1
– tuberosity K06.1

Enteritis, regional K50.8X

Epidermal thickening NEC L85.–

Epidermolysis bullosa
– acquired L12.3X
– dystrophica Q81.2X
– letalis Q81.1X
– simplex Q81.0X

Epilepsy G40.VX

Epiloia Q85.1X

Epistaxis R04.0

Epithelioma
– basal cell M8090/3
– malignant M8011/3
– NOS M8011/3

Epstein's pearl K09.83

Epulis
– congenital D10.33
– fibrous K06.82
– giant cell K06.81

Erosion of teeth K03.2
– due to
– – diet K03.22
– – drugs and medicaments K03.23
– – regurgitation, persistent K03.21
– – vomiting, persistent K03.21
– idiopathic K03.24
– occupational K03.20

Eruption
– cyst K09.00
– herpetiform K12.02
– varicelliform, Kaposi's B00.0X

Erythema
– infectiosum B08.3X
– multiforme L51.–
– – bullous L51.1X
– – nonbullous L51.0X

Erythraemia, acute M9841/3, C94.0X

Erythroleukaemia C94.0X

Erythromycin, adverse effects Y40.3X

Erythroplakia K13.22

Erythroplasia, Queyrat's M8080/2

Ewing's sarcoma M9260/3

Exarticulation of tooth S03.22

Exfoliation of teeth, due to systemic causes E08.0X

Exostosis K10.88

Extrusion of tooth S03.21

Eyelid
– open wound S01.1
– superficial injury S00.2

Fabry(–Anderson) disease E75.20

Face, facial
– bones, fracture S02.–
– congenital malformations NEC Q18.–
– injury, crushing S07.0
– pain NOS R51.X1

Facies, compression Q67.1

Factor VIII deficiency, hereditary D66.XX

Factor IX deficiency, hereditary D67.XX

Factor XI deficiency, hereditary D68.1X

Fallot's tetralogy Q21.3X

Fasciculation R25.3

Fasciitis, nodular M72.3X

Felty's syndrome M05.VX

Fetal alcohol syndrome Q86.0X

Fever
– arthropod-borne viral A93.8
– glandular B27.8X
– Indiana A93.8X

– scarlet A38.XX
– spotted A77.VX
– typhus A75.VX
– uveoparotid D86.8X

Fibrolipoma M8851/0

Fibroma
– ameloblastic M9330/0
– cementifying M9274/0
– chondromyxoid M9241/0
– desmoplastic M8823/1
– invasive M8821/1
– molle M8851/0
– NOS M8810/0
– odontogenic
– – central M9321/0
– – peripheral M9322/0
– ossifying M9262/0

Fibromatosis
– aggressive M8821/1
– gingival K06.10
– pseudosarcomatous M72.4X

Fibromyoma M8890/0

Fibromyxoma M8811/0

Fibromyxosarcoma M8811/3

Fibro-odontoma, ameloblastic M9290/0

Fibro-osteoma M9262/0

Fibrosarcoma
– ameloblastic M9330/3
– NOS M8810/3
– odontogenic M9330/3
– periosteal M8812/3

Fibrosis
– cystic E84.VX
– oral submucous K13.5

Fibroxanthoma M8830/0

Fifth disease B08.3X

Filariasis B74.VX

Findings, abnormal
– saliva R85.XX
– skull and head, on diagnostic imaging, NEC R93.0

Fistula (of)
– branchial cleft Q18.0
– lip, congenital Q38.00
– oral K13.71
– persistent postoperative T81.8
– salivary gland K11.4
– – congenital Q38.43

Flabby ridge K06.84

Fluorosis, dental K00.30

Flushing R23.2

Folate deficiency anaemia D52.VX

Follicle, thickened K05.33

Food
– hot, self-harm X77.VX
– toxic effect of noxious substances NEC T62

Foot and mouth disease B08.8X

Fordyce
– condition Q38.60
– disease Q38.60

Foreign
– body
– – granuloma, of face L92.3X
– – in alimentary tract T18.–
– – in mouth T18.0

Fracture (*continued*)
- tooth (*continued*)
- - crown (*continued*)
- - - without pulpal involvement S02.51
- - - with pulpal involvement S02.52
- - enamel S02.50
- - multiple S02.57
- - root S02.53
- vault S02.0
- zygoma S02.41

Frenulum, malignant neoplasm
- lingual C00.2X
- lower lip C00.4X
- upper lip C00.3X

Fröhlich's syndrome E23.61

Frostbite
- sequelae T95.0
- superficial
- - head T33.0
- - multiple regions T35.0
- - neck T33.1
- with tissue necrosis
- - head T34.0
- - multiple regions T35.1
- - neck T34.1

Fumes, NEC, toxic effect T59

Furrows
- circumoral A50.50
- Parrot's A50.50

Furuncle
- face L02.0
- neck L02.1

Fusion of teeth K00.23

Galactosaemia E74.2X

Gangrene, gangrenous
- fusospirochaetal A69.0
- pulpal K04.1
- stomatitis A69.0

Gases
– therapeutic
– – adverse effects Y48.–
– – poisoning T41
– NEC, toxic effect T59

Gaucher's disease E75.21

Gemination of teeth K00.23

Geographic
– stomatitis K12.11
– tongue K14.1

Geotrichosis B48.3X

German measles B06.8X

Giant cell
– arteritis M31.6X
– epulis K06.81
– granuloma
– – central K10.1
– – NOS K10.1
– – peripheral K06.81

Giant urticaria T78.3

Gigantism, pituitary E22.01

Gingiva, gingival
– carcinoma in situ D00.02
– cyst
– – developmental odontogenic K09.01
– – of adult K06.80
– – of newborn K09.82
– enlargement K06.1
– fibromatosis K06.10
– lesions due to
– – toothbrushing K06.21
– – traumatic occlusion K06.20
– neoplasm
– – benign D10.33
– – malignant C03.–

Gingiva, gingival (*continued*)
– recession K06.0
– – generalized K06.01
– – localized K06.00
– – postinfective K06.0
– – postoperative K06.0

Gingivitis
– acute K05.0
– – ulcerative, necrotizing A69.10
– associated with menstrual cycle N94.8X
– chronic K05.1
– – desquamative K05.13
– – hyperplastic K05.11
– – ulcerative K05.12
– – – necrotizing A69.10
– fusospirochaetal A69.10
– pregnancy O26.80
– Vincent's A69.10

Gingivostomatitis
– herpesviral B00.2X
– streptococcal, acute K05.00

Glanders A24.–

Glands, swollen, head and neck R59.VX

Glandular fever B27.8X

Glomangioma M8712/0

Glossitis K14.0
– areata exfoliativa K14.1
– atrophic NOS K14.42
– median rhomboid K14.2
– migratory, benign K14.1
– syphilitic A52.72

Glossodynia K14.69

Glossopyrosis K14.60

Glucocorticoids, topical, poisoning T49

Glycogen storage disease E74.0X

Goldenhar's syndrome Q87.01

Gonococcus, gonococcal (infection)
– stomatitis A54.8X
– temporomandibular joint A54.4X M01.3

Granuloma, granulomatous
– annulare L92.0X
– apical K04.5X
– candidal, oral B37.05
– disease, chronic (childhood) D71.XX
– eosinophilic D76.00
– – of oral mucosa K13.41
– – of skin L92.2X
– faciale L92.2X
– foreign body L92.3X
– giant cell
– – central K10.1
– – NOS K10.1
– – peripheral K06.81
– gravidarum O26.81
– Hodgkin's M9661/3
– inguinale A58.XX
– internal K03.31
– lethal midline M31.2
– pregnancy O26.81
– pulse K10.23
– pyogenic, of
– – face L98.0X
– – gingiva K06.83
– – oral mucosa K13.40

Granulomatosis
– respiratory, necrotizing M31.3X
– Wegener's M31.3X

Grawitz' tumour M8312/3

Growth hormone deficiency, idiopathic E23.01

Gumma (syphilitic) (of)
– oral tissues A52.70
– yaws A66.4X

Haemangioendothelioma
– benign M9130/0
– malignant M9130/3
– NOS M9130/1

Haemangioma M9120/0, D18.0X
– capillary M9131/0
– cavernous M9121/0

Haemangiopericytoma
– benign M9150/0
– malignant M9150/3
– NOS M9150/1

Haematoma, complicating a procedure, NEC T81.0

Haemochromatosis E83.1X

Haemolymphangioma M9175/0

Haemorrhage, haemorrhagic (of)
– complicating a procedure, NEC T81.0
– condition, NOS D69.9X
– disorder, due to circulating anticoagulants D68.3X
– respiratory passages R04.–
– throat R04.1

Hailey–Hailey disease Q82.80

Hairy
– leukoplakia K13.3X
– tongue, due to antibiotics K14.38

Halitosis R19.6

Hallucinogens
– poisoning T40
– self-poisoning X62.–

Hand, foot and mouth disease B08.4

Hand–Schüller–Christian disease D76.01

Head
– abnormal finding, diagnostic imaging R93.0
– blood vessels, injury NEC S09.0
– burn, with burn of neck T20.–
– – first degree T20.1
– – second degree T20.2
– – sequelae T95.0
– – third degree T20.3
– corrosion, with corrosion of neck T20.–
– – first degree T20.5
– – second degree T20.6
– – sequelae T95.0
– – third degree T20.7
– frostbite
– – sequelae T95.0
– – superficial T33.0
– – with tissue necrosis T34.0
– injury
– – crushing S07.–
– – multiple S09.7
– – NOS S09.9
– – superficial S00.–
– – – multiple S00.7
– – – sequelae T90.–
– – – with superficial injury of neck T00.0
– movements, abnormal R25.0
– muscle, injury S09.1
– neoplasm, malignant, NOS C76.0
– swelling, mass and lump, localized R22.0
– tendon, injury S09.1
– wound, open S01.–
– – multiple S01.7
– – – sequelae T90.–
– – with open wound of neck T01.0

Headache NOS R51.X0

Heat, effects of T67

Heerfordt's syndrome D86.8X

Helminthiasis B83.VX

Hemiatrophy of tongue K14.82

Hemihypertrophy of tongue K14.81

Herpangina B08.5X

Herpes, herpetic
- eczema B00.0
- gingivostomatitis B00.2X
- pharyngotonsillitis B00.2
- simplex
- – facialis B00.10
- – labialis B00.11
- whitlow B00.8X
- zoster B02.–
- – postherpetic neuralgia B02.2 G53.0

Histiocytoma, fibrous
- malignant M8830/3
- NOS M8830/1

Histiocytosis
- Langerhans' cell D76.0
- malignant M9720/3
- syndrome NEC D76.3X
- X (chronic) D76.0
- Y K13.42

Histoplasmosis B39.VX

HIV disease (*see* Human immunodeficiency virus disease)

Hodgkin's
- disease M9650/3, C81.VX
- granuloma M9661/3

Hookworm disease B76.VX

Hormone(s) NEC
- adverse effects Y42.–
- antagonists
- – adverse effects Y42.–
- – poisoning T38
- poisoning T38
- synthetic substitutes
- – adverse effects Y42.–
- – poisoning T38

Horner's syndrome G90.2X

Human immunodeficiency virus disease
- NOS B24.XX
- resulting in
- - bacterial infection B20.1X
- - Burkitt's lymphoma B21.1X
- - candidiasis B20.4X
- - cytomegaloviral disease B20.2X
- - HIV infection syndrome, acute B23.0X
- - infectious disease B20.-
- - Kaposi's sarcoma B21.0X
- - lymphadenopathy, generalized (persistent) B23.1X
- - malignant neoplasms B21.-
- - - multiple B21.7X
- - multiple infections B20.7X
- - mycobacterial infection B20.0X
- - mycosis B20.5X
- - non-Hodgkin's lymphoma B21.2X
- - parasitic disease B20.-
- - tuberculosis B20.0X
- - viral infection B20.3X

Hurler's syndrome E76.VX

Hutchinson's
- incisors A50.51
- melanotic freckle M8742/2

Hydantoin derivatives, adverse effects Y46.2X

Hydrocarbons, toxic effect T53

Hygroma, cystic M9173/0

Hyperaemia K04.00

Hyperaesthesia of skin R20.3

Hyperalimentation NEC E67.-

Hypercarotenaemia E67.1X

Hypercementosis K03.4
- in Paget's disease M88.-

Hypergammaglobulinaemia, hypergammaglobulinaemic
– polyclonal D89.0X
– purpura, benign D89.0X

Hypernephroma M8312/3

Hyperostosis
– cortical, infantile M89.80
– of skull M85.2

Hyperparathyroidism
– NOS E21.3X
– primary E21.0X
– secondary NEC E21.1X

Hyperpigmentation, melanin, NEC L81.4X

Hyperplasia (of)
– denture K06.23
– focal epithelial B07.X2
– irritative of
– – edentulous alveolar ridge K06.23
– – oral mucosa K13.6
– mandible K07.01
– – unilateral condylar
– maxilla K07.00
– palate, papillary K12.13

Hypersecretion K11.72

Hypersensitivity NOS T78.4

Hypertelorism (ocular) Q75.2

Hypertrophy
– hemifacial Q67.42
– salivary gland K11.1
– tongue K14.81
– – papillae K14.3
– – – foliate K14.32

Hypervitaminosis D E67.3X

Hypnotic drugs (*see* Sedative–hypnotic drugs)

Hypoaesthesia of skin R20.1

Hypochondroplasia Q77.4X

Hypodontia K00.00

Hypogammaglobulinaemia D80.VX

Hypoparathyroidism E20.VX

Hypophosphatasia E83.30

Hypopituitarism E23.0

Hypoplasia (of)
- cementum K00.43
- enamel K00.40
- - neonatal K00.42
- - prenatal K00.41
- mandible K07.04
- - unilateral condylar K10.82
- maxilla K07.03
- tongue Q38.36

Ichthyosis, congenital Q87.VX

Idiosyncracy NOS T78.4

Imbrication K07.30

Immunodeficiency
- with antibody defects D80.VX
- with defects NEC D82.–

Immunosuppressive agents, adverse effects Y43.4X

Impacted tooth, teeth K01.1
- abnormal position K07.35
- maxillary
- - canine K01.12
- - incisor K01.10
- - molar K01.16
- - premolar K01.14
- mandibular
- - canine K01.13

Impacted tooth, teeth K01.1 (*continued*)
- mandibular (*continued*)
- - incisor K01.11
- - molar K01.17
- - premolar K01.15
- normal position K01.1
- supernumerary K01.18

Incisors
- conical K00.25
- Hutchinson's A50.51
- peg-shaped K00.25
- shovel-shaped K00.25
- T-shaped K00.25

Incontinentia pigmenti Q82.3X

Indiana fever A93.8X

Infection (of)
- due to
- - fixation device, internal T84.6
- - HIV disease B20.–
- - - bacterial B20.1X
- - - multiple B20.7X
- - - mycobacterial B20.0X
- - - viral B20.3X
- - joint prosthesis, internal T84.5
- - orthopaedic devices, implants and grafts, internal T84.7
- gonococcal A54.–
- - of temporomandibular joint A54.4X M01.3
- meningococcal A39.VX
- mycetoma B47.VX
- mycobacterial A31.8
- - due to HIV disease B20.0X
- orthopoxvirus B08.0
- postprocedural, NEC T81.4
- skin, local, NEC L08.–
- spirochaetal A69.–
- subcutaneous tissue, local, NEC L08.–
- Vincent's A69.10

Inflammatory reaction due to
- fixation device, internal T84.6
- joint prosthesis, internal T84.5
- orthopaedic devices, implants and grafts, internal T84.7

Influenza
– virus identified J10.1X
– virus not identified J11.1X

Injury (of)
– blood vessels
– – head NEC S09.0
– – neck S15.–
– cranial nerves
– – fifth S04.3
– – ninth S04.80
– – sequelae T90.–
– – seventh S04.5
– – twelfth S04.81
– crushing
– – face S07.0
– – head S07.–
– – – and neck T04.0
– – skull S07.1
– superficial
– – cheek, internal S00.50
– – ear S00.4
– – eyelid S00.2
– – head S00.–
– – – and neck T00.0
– – – multiple
– – – sequelae T90.–
– – lip S00.52
– – mouth S00.51
– – multiple body regions T00.–
– – neck S10.VX
– – nose S00.3
– – periocular S00.2
– – scalp S00.0
– – tongue S00.51

Insufficiency, adrenocortical, primary E27.1

Intrusion of tooth S03.21

Jaundice NOS R17.XX

Jaw
– abnormal closure K07.50

Jaw (*continued*)
- alveolitis K10.3
- asymmetry K07.10
- clicking (snapping) K07.61
- cyst K09.–
- disease NEC K10.–
- dislocation S03.0
- inflammatory condition K10.2
- osteitis K10.20
- osteomalacia, adult M83.VX
- osteomyelitis K10.21
- – syphilitic A52.73
- osteoporosis
- – without pathological fracture M81.VX
- – with pathological fracture M80.VX
- Paget's disease M88.8
- periostitis K10.22
- – chronic K10.23
- tuberculosis A18.00 M01.1

Jaw-winking syndrome Q07.8X

Kaposi's
- sarcoma M9140/3
- – due to HIV disease B21.0X
- – lymph nodes, cervicofacial C46.3X
- – palate C46.2
- – skin, facial C46.0X
- – soft tissue, oral C46.1X
- varicelliform eruption B00.0X

Kawasaki's syndrome M30.3X

Kelly–Paterson syndrome D50.1X

Keloid scar L91.0X

Keratoacanthoma L85.8X

Keratocyst K09.02

Keratosis
- actinic (senile) (solar) L57.0
- follicularis Q82.81

– frictional K06.22
– functional K06.22
– palmaris et plantaris, inherited Q82.82
– seborrheic L82.XX

Klinefelter's syndrome Q98.V0

Klippel–Feil syndrome Q76.1

Koplik's spots B05.8X

Kwashiorkor E40.XX

Laceration, accidental, during a procedure, NEC T81.2

Langerhans' cell histiocytosis D76.0

Large cell (diffuse) non-Hodgkin's lymphoma C83.3X

Lead, toxic effect T56.0

Leiomyofibroma M8890/0

Leiomyoma D21.0
– NOS M8890/0
– vascular M8894/0

Leiomyosarcoma NOS M8890/3

Leishmaniasis, mucocutaneous B55.2X

Lentigo L81.4X
– maligna M8742/2

Leprosy A30.VX

Lesch–Nyhan syndrome E79.1X

Letterer–Siwe disease M9722/3, C96.0X

Leukaemia
– acute M9801/3
– aleukaemic M9804/3
– chronic M9803/3

Leukaemia (*continued*)
– lymphoid M9820/3, C91.VX
– monocytic M9890/3, C93.VX
– myeloid M9860/3, C92.VX
– NOS M9800/3, C95.VX

Leukoderma NEC L81.5X

Leukoedema K13.23

Leukokeratosis
– nicotina palati K13.24
– oris Q38.61

Leukoplakia
– candidal B37.02
– hairy K13.3X
– idiopathic K13.20
– tobacco-associated K13.21

Lichen, lichenoid
– drug reaction L43.2X
– planus L43.–
– – atrophic and erosive L43.82
– – bullous L43.1X
– – papular L43.80
– – plaque type L43.83
– – reticular L43.81
– sclerosus et atrophicus L90.0X

Light, effects of T67

Linea alba K13.78

Lingua
– indentata K14.80
– villosa nigra K14.31

Lip(s)
– biting K13.1
– carcinoma in situ
– – skin D04.0
– – vermilion border D00.00
– fistula, congenital Q38.00

– malformation, congenital, NEC Q38.0
– melanoma in situ
– – skin D03.30
– – vermilion border D03.0X
– neoplasm
– – benign D10.0
– – malignant C00.–
– – – secondary C79.2X
– – – skin C44.0
– – – vermilion border (lipstick area) C00.–
– open wound S01.51
– overlapping lesion C00.8
– superficial injury S00.52

Lipidaemia NEC E78.–

Lipoma NOS M8850/0

Lipoprotein metabolism, disorder E78.8X

Liposarcoma NOS M8850/3

Lisping F80.8X

Lupus erythematosus
– discoid L93.0X
– systemic M32.VX

Luxation of tooth S03.20

Lymphadenitis
– acute L04.0
– chronic I88.1X

Lymphadenopathy
– cervical A28.11
– generalized (persistent), due to HIV disease B23.1X
– tuberculous, facial and cervical A18.2X

Lymphangioma M9170/0, D18.1X
– capillary M9170/0
– cavernous M9172/0
– cystic M9173/0

Lymphangiosarcoma M9170/3

Lymph node(s)
– enlarged R59.VX
– neoplasm
– – benign D36.0X
– – malignant C77.0
– syndrome, mucocutaneous M30.3X

Lymphoepithelioma M8082/3

Lymphogranuloma, chlamydial (venereum) A55.XX

Lymphoma
– Burkitt's M9687/3, C83.7X
– – due to HIV disease B21.1X
– malignant
– – follicular M969
– – nodular M969
– – NOS M9590/3
– non-Hodgkin's
– – diffuse C83.–
– – due to HIV disease B21.2X
– – follicular C82.VX
– – large cell (diffuse) C83.3X
– – nodular C82.VX
– – NOS M9591/3
– – T-cell, peripheral and cutaneous M970, C84.–

Lymphosarcoma NOS M9592/3, C85.0X

Macrocephaly Q75.3

Macrocheilia Q18.6

Macrodontia K00.20

Macroglobulinaemia, Waldenström's M9761/3, C88.0X

Macroglossia Q38.2

Macrognathism
– both jaws K07.02
– mandibular K07.01
– maxillary K07.00

Macrolides, adverse effects Y40.3X

Macrostomia Q18.4

Maffucci's syndrome Q78.4

Malformation, congenital (of)
– arteries Q25.–
– cardiac septa Q21.–
– endocrine glands Q89.2
– face Q18.–
– – bones NEC Q75.–
– lips NEC Q38.0
– mouth Q38.–
– musculoskeletal system NEC Q79.–
– neck Q18.–
– nervous system Q07.–
– nose Q30.–
– palate NEC Q38.5
– pharynx Q38.–
– salivary glands and ducts Q38.4
– skin NEC Q82.–
– skull bones NEC Q75.–
– spine Q76.–
– syndromes
– – affecting multiple systems Q87.–
– – associated with short stature Q87.1
– – due to known exogenous causes NEC Q86.–
– – involving early overgrowth Q87.3
– – involving limbs Q87.2
– thorax, bony Q76.–
– tongue Q38.–
– vascular system, peripheral Q27.–

Malocclusion (*see also* **Anomalies, dentofacial**)
– due to
– – abnormal swallowing K07.51
– mouth breathing K07.54
– tongue, lip or finger habits K07.55

Maple-syrup-urine disease E71.0X

Marasmus, nutritional E41.XX

Marble bone disease Q78.2X

Marcus Gunn's syndrome Q07.8X

Marfan's syndrome Q87.4X

Mast cell tumour D47.0X

Mastocytosis Q82.2

Materia alba K03.63

Maxillitis, neonatal K10.24

Measles B05.8X
– German B06.8X

Mediterranean anaemia D56.VX

Melanin
– hyperpigmentation NEC L81.4X
– pigmentation, excessive K13.70

Melanodontia, infantile K02.4

Melanodontoclasia K02.4

Melanoma
– amelanotic M8730/3
– balloon cell M8722/3
– in situ M8720/2
– – lip
– – – skin D03.30
– – – vermilion border D03.0X
– – mucosa
– – – labial D03.0X
– – – oral D03.8X
– – skin
– – – facial D03.31
– – – lip D03.30
– juvenile M8770/0
– malignant
– – in Hutchinson's melanotic freckle M8742/3
– – in junctional naevus M8740/3
– – in precancerous melanosis M8741/3
– – NOS M8720/3
– – skin
– – – face NOS C43.3
– – – lip C43.0
– – – overlapping C43.8

– spindle cell M8772/3
– superficial spreading M8743/3

Melanoplakia K13.70

Melanosis
– precancerous NOS M8741/2
– smoker's K13.70

Melioidosis A24.3X

Meningioma NOS M9530/0

Mercury, toxic effect T56.1

Mesenchymoma, malignant M8990/3

Mesio-occlusion K07.21

Mesiodens K00.10

Metabolism, disorder
– calcium E83.5X
– carbohydrate E74
– galactose E74.2X
– iron E83.1
– mineral E83.–
– phosphorus E83.3
– zinc E83.2

Metals, toxic effect T56

Microangiopathy, hyaline K10.23

Microcheilia Q18.7

Microdontia K00.21

Microglossia Q38.35

Micrognathism
– both jaws K07.05
– mandibular K07.04
– maxillary K07.03

Microstomia Q18.5

Midline deviation K07.26

Migraine G43.VX

Mikulicz'
– aphthae K12.00
– disease K11.81

Misadventure during surgical and medical care
– cut, puncture, perforation or haemorrhage,
    unintentional Y60.0
– foreign body accidentally left in body Y61.0
– NEC Y65.8

Moebius' syndrome Q87.02

Molars, mulberry A50.52

Molluscum contagiosum B08.1X

Moniliasis B37.–

Mononucleosis, infectious B27.8X

Morphea L94.0X

Morquio's syndrome E76.VX

Motor neuron disease G12.2

Mottling, enamel
– endemic (fluoride) K00.30
– non-endemic K00.31

Mouth
– breathing R06.5
– burn, with burn of pharynx T28.0
– corrosion, with corrosion of pharynx T28.5
– dry NOS R68.2
– floor
– – carcinoma in situ D00.04
– – neoplasm

– – – benign D10.2
– – – malignant C04.–
– open wound S01.50
– superficial injury S00.51

Movements, abnormal
– head R25.0
– involuntary R25.–

Mucinosis, focal oral K13.73

Mucocele
– maxillary sinus J34.1X
– salivary gland K11.6

Mucocutaneous lymph node syndrome M30.3X

Mucormycosis B46.5X

Mulberry molars A50.52

Mumps B26.9X

Muscle
– calcification M61.VX
– disorder NEC M62.VX
– ossification M61.VX
– sternocleidomastoid, congenital deformity Q68.0

Myalgia M79.1X

Mycetoma infection B47.VX

Mycobacterium, **mycobacterial**
– *chelonei* A31.81
– infection A31.8
– – due to HIV disease B20.0X
– *intracellulare* A31.80

Mycosis
– due to HIV disease B20.5X
– fungoides M9700/3, C84.0X
– NEC B48.–

Myeloma
– multiple M9732/3, C90.0X
– solitary C90.2X

Myelomatosis M9732/3

Myiasis B87.8X

Myoblastoma, granular cell M9580/0

Myoepithelioma M8982/0

Myofibroma M8890/0

Myokymia, facial G51.4

Myositis ossificans M61.VX

Myxofibroma, odontogenic M9320/0

Myxoma
– jaw M9320/0
– NOS M8840/0
– odontogenic M9320/0

Myxosarcoma M8840/3

Naevus
– blue
– – cellular M8790/0 D22.–
– – malignant M8780/3 C43.–
– – NOS M8780/0 D22.–
– compound M8760/0 D22.–
– dermal M8750/0 D22.–
– epithelioid and spindle cell M8770/0 D22.–
– epithelioid cell M8771/0 D22.–
– flammeus Q82.5X
– intradermal M8750/0 D22.–
– intraepidermal M8740/0 D22.–
– junction, junctional M8740/0 D22.–
– juvenile M8770/0 D22.–
– melanocytic
– – face NOS D22.3
– – lip D22.0

– non-neoplastic, congenital Q82.5X
– nonpigmented M8730/0 D22.–
– pigmented NOS M8720/0 D22.–
– portwine Q82.5X
– sanguineous Q82.5X
– spindle cell M8772/0 D22.–
– vascular NOS Q82.5X
– verrucous Q82.5X
– white sponge Q38.61

Narcotics
– poisoning T40
– self-poisoning X62.–

Neck
– blood vessels, injury S15.–
– burn, with burn of head T20.–
– – first degree T20.1
– – second degree T20.2
– – sequelae T95.0
– – third degree T20.3
– congenital malformations NEC Q18.–
– corrosion, with corrosion of head T20.–
– – first degree T20.5
– – second degree T20.6
– – sequelae T95.0
– – third degree T20.7
– frostbite
– – superficial T33.1
– – with tissue necrosis T34.1
– neoplasm, malignant C76.0
– open wound S11.VX
– – with open wound of head T01.0
– superficial injury S10.VX
– – with superficial injury of head T00.0
– swelling, mass and lump, localized R22.1
– webbing of Q18.3

Necrosis, pulp K04.1

Neoplasm
– benign (of)
– – alveolar ridge D10.33
– – bone and cartilage D16.–

Neoplasm (*continued*)
– benign (of) (*continued*)
– – bone and cartilage (*continued*)
– – – mandible D16.50
– – – maxilla D16.40
– – commissure, buccal mucosal D10.31
– – connective tissue, head, face and neck D21.0
– – gingiva D10.33
– – hypopharynx D10.7
– – lip(s)
– – – labial mucosa D10.07
– – – vermilion border D10.06
– – – – with labial mucosa D10.08
– – – lower
– – – – labial mucosa D10.04
– – – – vermilion border D10.03
– – – – – with labial mucosa D10.05
– – – upper
– – – – labial mucosa D10.01
– – – – vermilion border D10.00
– – – – – with labial mucosa D10.02
– – lipomatous, head, face and neck D17.0
– – lymph nodes, head and neck D36.0X
– – mouth, floor D10.2
– – mucosa
– – – buccal D10.30
– – – labial D10.07
– – – – lower D10.04
– – – – upper D10.01
– – nasopharynx D10.6
– – nerves
– – – cranial D33.3
– – – peripheral, head and neck D36.1X
– – odontogenic tissues D16.–
– – – mandible D16.51
– – – maxilla D16.41
– – oropharynx NEC D10.5
– – palate
– – – hard D10.34
– – – soft D10.35
– – pharynx NOS D10.9
– – retromolar area D10.37
– – salivary gland
– – – major D11.–
– – – minor NOS D10.3

– – – parotid D11.0
– – – sublingual D11.71
– – – submandibular D11.70
– – sinuses D14.0X
– – skin
– – – face NOS D23.3
– – – lip D23.0
– – sulcus, buccal D10.32
– – tongue
– – – base D10.10
– – – borders D10.12
– – – dorsal surface D10.11
– – – tip D10.12
– – – tonsil D10.14
– – – ventral surface D10.13
– – tonsil, tonsillar D10.4
– – – fossa D10.5
– – – lingual D10.14
– – – pillar D10.5
– – tuberosity D10.38
– – uvula D10.36
– malignant (of)
– – bone and articular cartilage C41.–
– – – overlapping lesion C41.8
– – branchial cleft C10.4
– – commissure, labial C00.6
– – connective tissue, head, face and neck C49.0
– – due to HIV disease B21.–
– – face, facial
– – – bone, secondary NOS C79.59
– – – NOS C76.0
– – – secondary C79.2X
– – frenulum
– – – labial
– – – – lower C00.4X
– – – – upper C00.3X
– – – lingual C02.2X
– – gingiva C03.–
– – – mandible C03.1X
– – – maxilla C03.0X
– – gum
– – – lower C03.1X
– – – upper C03.0X
– – haematopoietic tissue C96.–
– – head NOS C76.0

Neoplasm (*continued*)
– malignant (of) (*continued*)
– – lip
– – – frenulum C00.4
– – – – lower C00.4X
– – – – upper C00.3X
– – – overlapping lesion C00.8
– – – secondary C79.2X
– – – skin C44.0
– – – vermilion border (lipstick area)
– – – – lower C00.1X
– – – – NOS C00.2X
– – – – upper C00.0X
– – lymph nodes, head, face and neck C77.0
– – lymphoid tissue C96.–
– – mandible, mandibular
– – – alveolar ridge mucosa C03.1X
– – – gingiva C03.1X
– – – intraosseous salivary gland tumour C41.12
– – – odontogenic tumour C41.11
– – – retromolar area C06.21
– – – sarcoma C41.10
– – – secondary C79.51
– – maxilla, maxillary
– – – alveolar ridge mucosa C03.0X
– – – carcinoma C41.01
– – – gingiva C03.0X
– – – intraosseous salivary gland tumour C41.02
– – – odontogenic tumour C41.01
– – – sarcoma C41.00
– – – secondary C79.50
– – – tuberosity C06.20
– – mouth
– – – floor C04.–
– – – – anterior C04.0
– – – – lateral C04.1
– – – – overlapping C04.8
– – – overlapping lesion C06.8
– – – retromolar area C06.2
– – – – mandibular C06.21
– – – vestibule C06.1
– – mucosa
– – – alveolar ridge
– – – – mandibular C03.1X
– – – – maxillary C03.0X

– – – buccal C06.0
– – – labial
– – – – lower C00.4X
– – – – NOS C00.5X
– – – – upper C00.3X
– – multiple sites C97.–
– – nasopharynx C11.–
– – – anterior wall C11.3
– – – posterior wall C11.1
– – neck NOS C76.0
– – nerves
– – – cranial C72.5X
– – – peripheral, head, face and neck C47.0
– – nose, nasal
– – – cavity C30.0
– – oropharynx C10.–
– – – lateral wall C10.2
– – – overlapping lesion C10.8
– – – posterior wall C10.3
– – palate C05.–
– – – hard C05.0
– – – overlapping C05.8
– – – soft C05.1
– – – – nasopharyngeal surface C11.3X
– – parotid gland C07.XX
– – plasma cell C90.–
– – salivary gland
– – – major C08.–
– – – overlapping lesion C08.8
– – – parotid C07.XX
– – – sublingual C08.1
– – – submandibular C08.0
– – – submaxillary C08.0
– – sinus
– – – accessory NOS C31.9
– – – – overlapping lesion C31.8
– – – ethmoidal C31.1
– – – frontal C31.2
– – – maxillary C31.0
– – – sphenoidal C31.3
– – skin NEC
– – – face NOS C44.3
– – – lip C44.0
– – – overlapping lesion C44.8

Neoplasm (*continued*)
– malignant (of) (*continued*)
– – tongue
– – – anterior two-thirds C02.3
– – – – dorsal surface C02.0X
– – – – ventral surface C02.2X
– – – base, dorsal surface C01
– – – border, lateral C02.11
– – – frenulum C02.2X
– – – overlapping lesion C02.8
– – – secondary C79.8X
– – – tip C02.10
– – – tonsil C02.4
– – tonsil, tonsillar
– – – fossa C09.0
– – – lingual C02.4
– – – palatine C09.9
– – – pillar C09.1
– – uvula C05.2
– – vallecula C10.0
– metastatic M8000/6
– uncertain or unknown behaviour
– – bone and articular cartilage D48.0X
– – connective tissue D48.1X
– – haematopoietic tissue D47.–
– – lip D37.0
– – lymphoid tissue D47.–
– – nerves
– – – cranial D43.3
– – – peripheral D48.2X
– – oral cavity D37.0
– – pharynx D37.0
– – salivary gland
– – – major D37.00
– – – minor D37.01
– – sinus
– – – maxillary D38.50
– – – NEC D38.51
– – skin D48.5X

Neuralgia
– glossopharyngeal G52.1X
– head and neck NOS M79.2X
– postherpetic (postzoster) B02.2 G53.0

– – cranial nerve NEC G53.01
– – trigeminal G53.00
– trigeminal G50.0

Neurilemmoma
– malignant M9560/3
– NOS M9560/0

Neuritis, head and neck, NOS M79.2X

Neuroblastoma NOS M9500/3

Neurofibroma
– melanotic M9541/0
– NOS M9540/0
– plexiform M9550/0

Neurofibromatosis
– nonmalignant Q85.0X
– NOS M9540/1

Neurofibrosarcoma M9540/3

Neuroma NOS M9570/0

Neutropenia
– cyclic (periodic) D70.X1
– drug-induced D70.X2
– NOS D70.X3

Neutrophils, functional disorder D71.XX

Niacin deficiency E52.XX

Nicotine, toxic effect T65.2

Niemann–Pick disease E75.22

Nocardiosis A43.8X

Nodules, subcutaneous (localized) (superficial) R22.–

Noma A69.0

Non-Hodgkin's lymphoma
– diffuse, large cell C83.3X
– follicular C82.VX
– malignant NOS M9591/3
– nodular C82.VX

Noonan's syndrome Q87.1X

Nose, nasal
– anomalies associated with jaw anomalies Q30.8
– burn and corrosion T20.–
– cavity, malignant neoplasm C30.0
– congenital malformations NEC Q30.8
– dislocation S03.1
– fracture S02.2
– open wound S01.2
– sprain and strain S03.4
– superficial injury S00.3

Nutrient element deficiency NEC E61.VX

Occlusion, posterior lingual, of mandibular teeth K07.27

Odontoameloblastoma M9311/0

Odontoclasia K02.4

Odontodysplasia (regional) K00.45

Odontoma
– complex M9282/0
– compound M9281/0
– dilated K00.25
– fibroameloblastic M9290/0

Odontosarcoma, ameloblastic M9290/3

Oedema
– angioneurotic T78.3
– Quincke's T78.3

Oligodontia K00.00

Ollier's disease Q78.4

Oncocytoma M8290/0

Openbite K07.24

Opioids, adverse effects Y45.0X

Orf B08.00

Oro-facial-digital syndrome Q87.03

Orthopoxvirus infection B08.0

Ossification of muscle M61.VX

Osteitis (of)
– alveolar K10.3
– deformans M88.–
– jaw K10.20

Osteoarthritis/osteoarthrosis, temporomandibular joint M19.0X

Osteoblastoma M9200/0

Osteochondrodysplasia Q77.–

Osteochondroma M9210/0

Osteofibroma M9262/0

Osteogenesis imperfecta Q78.0X
– dental changes in K00.51

Osteoma
– NOS M9180/0
– osteoid NOS M9191/0

Osteomalacia, adult, of jaws M83.VX

Osteomyelitis (of)
– jaw K10.21
– – syphilitic A52.73
– maxilla, neonatal K10.24

Osteopetrosis Q78.2X

Osteophyte, temporomandibular joint K07.65

Osteopoikilosis Q78.8

Osteoporosis of jaws
– without pathological fracture M81.VX
– with pathological fracture M80.VX

Osteoradionecrosis K10.26

Osteosarcoma
– chondroblastic M9181/3
– fibroblastic M9182/3
– in Paget's disease of bone M9184/3
– juxtacortical M9190/3
– NOS M9180/3
– parosteal M9190/3
– telangiectatic M9183/3

Overbite
– excessive K07.23
– horizontal K07.22
– vertical K07.23

Overdose (*see* **Poisoning**)

Overjet, excessive K07.22

Oxycephaly Q75.02

Paget's disease
– facial bones M88.88
– mandible M88.81
– maxilla M88.80
– skull M88.0

Pain
– chest R07.–
– facial
– – atypical G50.1
– – NOS R51.X1
– temporomandibular joint NEC K07.63
– throat R07.0

Palate, palatal
– carcinoma in situ D00.03
– cleft Q35.–
– – hard

– – – bilateral Q35.2
– – – unilateral Q35.1
– – – with cleft lip
– – – – bilateral Q37.0
– – – – unilateral Q37.1
– – hard and soft
– – – bilateral Q35.4
– – – unilateral Q35.5
– – – with cleft lip
– – – – bilateral Q37.4
– – – – unilateral Q37.5
– – medial Q35.6
– – soft
– – – bilateral Q35.2
– – – unilateral Q35.3
– – – with cleft lip
– – – – bilateral Q37.2
– – – – unilateral Q37.3
– congenital malformations NEC Q38.5
– high arched Q38.51
– hyperplasia (papillary) K12.13
– neoplasm
– – benign
– – – hard D10.34
– – – soft D10.35
– – malignant
– – – hard C05.0
– – – soft C05.1
– perforation, due to syphilis A52.71
– smoker's K13.24

Palsy
– Bell's G51.0
– facial NEC G51.01

Papilloma
– inverted M8053/0
– keratotic M8052/0
– NOS M8050/0
– squamous (cell) M8052/0
– verrucous M8051/0

Papillomatosis NOS M8060/0

Paracoccidioidomycosis B41.VX

Paraesthesia of skin R20.2

Paraganglioma, carotid body M8692/1

Parageusia R43.2

Parathyroid gland disorder NEC E21.–

Parrot's furrows A50.50

Patent ductus arteriosus Q25.0X

Pellagra E52.XX

Pemphigoid
– bullous L12.0X
– cicatricial L12.1X
– mucous membrane, benign L12.1X

Pemphigus
– benign familial Q82.80
– drug-induced L10.5X
– foliaceus L10.2X
– vegetans L10.1X
– vulgaris L10.0X

Penicillins, adverse effects Y40.0X

Perforation, syphilitic, of palate A52.71

Periadenitis mucosa necrotica recurrens K12.01

Pericoronitis
– acute K05.22
– chronic K05.32

Periodontitis
– acute K05.2
– – apical
– – – NOS K04.41
– – – of pulpal origin K04.4
– chronic
– – apical K04.5X

– – complex K05.31
– – simplex K05.30

Periodontosis K05.4

Periostitis of jaw K10.22
– chronic K10.23

Perlèche NEC K13.00

Peroxidase defects E80.3

Pesticides, toxic effect T60

Petechiae R23.3X

Peutz–Jeghers syndrome Q85.80

Phaeochromocytoma
– malignant M8700/3
– NOS M8700/0

Phakomatoses NEC Q85.–

Pharyngitis, enteroviral vesicular B08.5

Pharyngotonsillitis, herpesviral B00.2

Phenylketonuria, classical E70.0X

Phlebolith I87.8X

Phlegmon of mouth K12.2

Pigmentation
– disorder NEC L81.–
– melanin, excessive K13.70

Pindborg tumour M9340/0

Pink spot K03.31

Pituitary gland
– disorder NEC E23.6

Pituitary gland (*continued*)
– hyperfunction E22.–
– hypofunction E23.0

Pityriasis rosea L42.XX

Plagiocephaly Q67.3

Plaque K03.66

Plasma cell tumour malignant, NOS C90.2

Plasmacytoma M9731/3 C90.2X

Platelet defects, qualitative D69.1X

Plummer–Vinson syndrome D50.1X

Poisoning (*see also* **individual drugs and drug types**)
– by agents primarily (acting on)
– – autonomic nervous system T44
– – cardiovascular system T46
– – gastrointestinal system T47
– – haematological T45
– – mucous membrane, topical T49
– – muscle T48
– – respiratory system T48
– – skin, topical T49
– – systemic T45

Polyarteritis nodosa M30.–

Polyarthrosis, temporomandibular joint M15.VX

Polycythaemia D75.VX
– vera M9950/1 D45.XX

Polyglandular dysfunction E31.VX

Polymorphonuclear neutrophils, functional disorder D71.XX

Polyp (of)
– maxillary sinus J33.8X
– pulpal K04.05

Porphyria, erythropoietic, hereditary E80.0X
– colour changes in teeth due to K00.82

Pregnancy
– excessive vomiting in O21.VX
– gingivitis O26.80
– granuloma O26.81
– related conditions NEC O26.8

Premolarization K00.26

Progeria E34.8X

Prognathism
– mandibular K07.11
– maxillary K07.12

Pseudarthrosis M84.1X

Pseudohypoparathyroidism E20.VX

Pseudoxanthoma elasticum Q82.84

Psoriasis
– pustular, generalized L40.1X
– vulgaris L40.0X

Psychodysleptics
– poisoning T40
– self-poisoning X62.–

Psychotropic drug NEC
– adverse effects Y49.9X
– poisoning T43

Pterygium colli Q18.3

Ptyalism K11.72

Pulp, pulpal
– abscess K04.02
– calcification K04.2
– degeneration K04.2
– diseases K04.–
– gangrene K04.1
– necrosis K04.1

Pulp, pulpal (*continued*)
– polyp K04.05
– stones K04.2

Pulpitis K04.0
– acute K04.01
– chronic K04.03
– – hyperplastic K04.05
– – ulcerative K04.04
– initial (hyperaemia) K04.00
– suppurative K04.02

Puncture, accidental, during a procedure, NEC T81.2

Purpura
– allergic D69.0X
– hypergammaglobulinaemic, benign D89.0X
– thrombocytopenic, idiopathic D69.3X

Pyoderma L08.0

Pyostomatitis vegetans L08.0X

Queyrat's erythroplasia M8080/2

Quinck's oedema T78.3

Radiation sickness T66

Ranula K11.6

Reiter's disease M02.3X

Renal failure, chronic N18.–

Rendu–Osler–Weber disease I78.0X

Resorption of teeth, pathological K03.3
– external K03.30
– internal K03.31

Retained dental root K08.3X

Reticulosarcoma M9593/3

Reticulum cell sarcoma C83.3X

Retinoblastoma NOS M9510/3

Retrognathism
– mandibular K07.13
– maxillary K07.14

Rhabdomyoma M8900/0

Rhabdomyosarcoma
– alveolar M8920/3
– embryonal M8910/3
– NOS M8900/3 D21.0

Rhinosporidiosis B48.1X

Riboflavin deficiency E53.0X

Rickets
– active E55.0X
– vitamin-D-resistant E83.31

Rickettsiosis, tick-borne A77.VX

Ridge, flabby K06.84

Riley–Day syndrome G90.1X

Robin's syndrome Q87.05

Rosacea L71.–

Rotation, tooth K03.32

Rubella B06.8X

Rupture of operation wound, NEC T81.3

Salicylates, adverse effects Y45.1X

Saliva, salivary
– duct
– – absence Q38.40

Saliva, salivary (*continued*)
– duct (*continued*)
– – accessory Q38.41
– – atresia Q38.42
– – calculus in K11.5X
– – fistula, congenital Q38.43
– – malformation, congenital Q38.4
– – stenosis K11.82
– – stone in K11.5X
– – stricture K11.82
– gland
– – abscess K11.3
– – absence Q38.40
– – accessory Q38.41
– – atresia Q38.42
– – atrophy K11.0
– – diseases K11.–
– – fistula K11.4
– – – congenital Q38.43
– – hypertrophy K11.1
– – lymphoepithelial lesion, benign K11.80
– – malformation, congenital Q38.4
– – neoplasm
– – – benign D11.–
– – – malignant C08.–
– hypersecretion K11.72
– hyposecretion K11.70
– secretion, disturbances K11.7

Sarcoidosis D86.8X

Sarcoma (of)
– alveolar soft part M9581/3
– ameloblastic M9330/3
– Ewing's M9260/3
– giant cell M8802/3
– – of bone M9250/3
– Kaposi's M9140/3
– – due to HIV disease B21.0X
– – lymph nodes, cervicofacial C46.3X
– – palate C46.2
– – skin, facial C46.0X
– – soft tissue, oral C46.1X
– myeloid M9930/3
– NOS M8800/3

– odontogenic M9270/3
– periosteal osteogenic M9190/3
– pleomorphic cell M8802/3
– reticulum cell C83.3X
– spindle cell M8801/3
– synovial NOS M9040/3

Scalp
– burn and corrosion T20.–
– open wound S01.0
– superficial injury S00.0

Scar, keloid L91.0X

Scarlet fever A38.XX

Scleroderma M34.VX
– linear, of face L94.1X
– localized, of face L94.0X

Sclerosis
– amyotrophic lateral G12.2X
– systemic M34.VX
– tuberous Q85.1X

Seafood, toxic effect of noxious substances T61

Sedative–hypnotic drugs, poisoning T42

Septicaemia, postprocedural T81.4

Sequelae (of)
– fracture, skull and facial bones T90.–
– injury
– – cranial nerves T90.–
– – eye and orbit T90.–
– – head T90.–

Sequestrum K10.25

Shell teeth K00.58

Shingles B02.–

Sialectasia K11.83

Sialoadenitis K11.2

Sialoadenopathy NOS K11.9

Sialolithiasis K11.5X

Sialometaplasia, necrotizing K11.85

Sialosis K11.84

Sicca syndrome M35.0X

Sickle-cell disorder D57.VX

Sickness, decompression T70.3

Simmonds' disease E23.00

Sinus (of)
− accessory
− − carcinoma in situ D02.3X
− − malignant neoplasm NOS C31.9
− barotrauma T70.1
− branchial cleft Q18.0
− maxillary
− − cyst and mucocele J34.1X
− − malignant neoplasm C31.0
− − polyp J33.8X
− neoplasm
− − benign D14.0X
− − malignant C31.−

Sinusitis
− acute J01.−
− − frontal J01.1
− − maxillary J01.0
− chronic J32.−
− − frontal J32.1
− − maxillary J32.0

Sjögren's syndrome M35.0X

Skin
− anaesthesia R20.0
− carcinoma in situ

Snoring R06.5

Soaps, toxic effect T55

Solvents, organic, toxic effect T52

Somatoform disorder F45.–

Soor NOS B37.09

Spacing, tooth K07.33

Spasm, clonic hemifacial G51.3

Speech
– articulation disorder F80.0
– disturbance NEC R47.–

Sporotrichosis B42.VX

Spot, spots
– café au lait L81.3X
– Koplik's B05.8X
– pink K03.31

Spotted fever A77.VX

Sprain (of)
– involving head and neck T03.0
– jaw S03.4

Stafne's cyst K10.02

Staining of teeth, intrinsic, NOS K00.8

Stammering F98.5

Steam, self-harm X77.–

Stevens–Johnson syndrome L51.1X

Stiffness, temporomandibular joint, NEC K07.64

Still's disease M08.VX

Stomatitis K12.–
– aphthous K12.00
– – cicatrizing K12.01
– artifacta K12.10
– candidal
– – acute
– – – erythematous (atrophic) B37.01
– – – pseudomembranous B37.00
– – chronic
– – – erythematous (atrophic) B37.03
– – – hyperplastic, multifocal-type B37.02
– contact K12.14
– cotton roll K12.14
– denture K12.11
– – candidal B37.03
– enteroviral vesicular B08.4X
– epizootic B08.8
– gangrenosa A69.0
– geographic K12.11
– gonococcal A54.8X
– herpetiformis K12.02
– nicotinic K13.24
– ulcerative, necrotizing A69.0
– vesicular
– – virus disease A93.8X
– – with exanthem B08.4X

Stone(s) (in)
– pulpal K04.2
– salivary duct K11.5X

Strain (of)
– involving head and neck T03.0
– jaw S03.4

Sturge–Weber(–Dimitri) syndrome Q85.81

Stuttering F98.5

Sulfonamides, adverse effects Y41.0X

Supernumerary teeth
– incisor and canine regions K00.10
– molar region K00.12
– premolar region K00.11

Supplementary teeth K00.1

Sutton's aphthae K12.01

Syndrome
- acquired immunodeficiency, NOS B24.XX
- Albers–Schönberg Q78.2X
- Albright(–McCune)(–Sternberg) Q78.1
- Apert's Q87.00
- cervical fusion Q76.1
- cri-du-chat Q93.4X
- defibrination D65.XX
- Di George's D82.1X
- Down's Q90.VX
- Edwards' Q91.3X
- Ehlers–Danlos Q79.6X
- Ellis–van Creveld Q77.6X
- Felty's M05.VX
- fetal alcohol Q86.0X
- Fröhlich's E23.61
- Goldenhar's Q87.01
- Heerfordt's D86.8X
- histiocytosis NEC D76.3X
- HIV infection, acute B23.0X
- Horner's G90.2X
- Hurler's E76.VX
- jaw-winking Q07.8X
- Kawasaki's M30.3X
- Kelly–Paterson D50.1X
- Klinefelter's Q98.V0
- Klippel–Feil Q76.1
- Lesch–Nyhan E79.1X
- lymph node, mucocutaneous M30.3X
- Maffucci's Q87.4
- Marcus Gunn's Q07.8X
- Marfan's Q87.4X
- Melkersson(–Rosenthal) G51.2X
- Moebius' Q87.02
- Morquio's E76.VX
- mucocutaneous lymph node M30.3X
- Noonan's Q87.1X
- oro-facial-digital Q87.03
- Patau's Q91.7X
- Peutz–Jeghers Q85.80
- Plummer–Vinson D50.1X
- Riley–Day G90.1X

Telangiectasia, haemorrhagic hereditary I78.0X

Temporomandibular joint
- arthritis
- - juvenile M08.VX
- - pyogenic M00.VX
- - rheumatoid M06.VX
- - - seropositive M05.VX
- - unspecified M13.9X
- arthropathy
- - postinfective M03.VX
- - reactive M02.3X
- - traumatic M12.5X
- arthrosis M19.0X
- disorder NEC K07.6
- gonococcal infection A54.4X M01.3
- osteoarthritis, osteoarthrosis M19.0X
- osteophyte K07.65
- pain NEC K07.63
- polyarthrosis M15.VX
- sprain and strain S03.4
- stiffness NEC K07.64
- tuberculosis A18.00
- villonodular synovitis (pigmented) M12.2X

Teratoma
- benign M9080/0
- malignant NOS M9080/3
- NOS M9080/1

Tetanus A35.XX

Tetracyclines, adverse effects Y40.4X
- colour changes in teeth due to K00.83

Tetralogy of Fallot Q21.3X

Thalassaemia D56.VX

Thiamine deficiency E51.–

Thickening, epidermal, NEC L85.–

Throat
- haemorrhage R04.1
- pain R07.0

Thrombocytopenia, thrombocytopenic
– NOS D69.6X
– purpura, idiopathic D69.3X

Thrush, oral, NOS B37.09

Thumb-sucking F98.8X

Thyroglossal
– cyst Q89.21
– duct, persistent Q89.20
– fistula Q89.22

Thyroid
– disorder NOS E07.9X
– lingual Q89.23

Tic douloureux G50.0

Tick-borne rickettsiosis A77.VX

Tinea
– barbae B35.0X
– capitis B35.0X

Tobacco, toxic effect T65.2

Tongue
– adhesion, congenital Q38.32
– atrophy K14.82
– – of papillae due to
– – – cleaning habits K14.40
– – – systemic conditions K14.41
– bifid Q38.31
– burning K14.60
– carcinoma in situ D00.06
– – ventral surface D00.05
– coated K14.30
– congenital malformations NEC Q38.–
– crenated K14.80
– diseases NEC K14.–
– epithelial disturbance K13.–
– fissured K14.5
– – congenital Q38.33

Tongue (*continued*)
– furrowed K14.5
– geographic K14.1
– hairy K14.31
– – black K14.31
– – due to antibiotics K14.38
– hemiatrophy K14.82
– hemihypertrophy K14.81
– hypertrophy K14.81
– – congenital Q38.34
– – of papillae K14.3
– hypoplasia Q38.36
– injury, superficial S00.51
– malformations, congenital, NEC Q38.–
– neoplasm
– – benign D10.1
– – malignant C02.–
– – – base, dorsal surface C01
– – – secondary C79.8X
– overlapping lesion C02.8
– painful NOS K14.69
– plicated K14.5
– scrotal K14.5
– tie Q38.1
– wound, open S01.50

Tonsil, tonsillar
– lingual
– – disease NEC K14.88
– – neoplasm
– – – benign D10.14
– – – malignant C02.4
– neoplasm
– – benign D10.–
– – malignant C09.–

Tonsillitis
– acute J03
– chronic J35.0

Tooth, teeth
– abnormalities, size and form K00.2
– abrasion K03.1
– – dentifrice K03.10
– – habitual K03.11

Tooth, teeth (*continued*)
– gemination K00.23
– grinding F45.82
– hard tissue
– – colour changes, posteruptive, due to
– – – betel-chewing K03.72
– – – metals, metallic compounds K03.70
– – – tobacco-chewing K03.72
– – diseases K03.–
– impacted
– – mandibular
– – – canine K01.13
– – – incisor K01.11
– – – molar K01.17
– – – premolar K01.15
– – maxillary
– – – canine K01.12
– – – incisor K01.10
– – – molar K01.16
– – – premolar K01.14
– – supernumerary K01.18
– intrusion S03.21
– loss due to accident, extraction or periodontal
  disease K08.1
– luxation S03.20
– mottled K00.3
– natal K00.60
– neonatal K00.61
– primary (deciduous)
– – premature shedding K00.65
– – retained (persistent) K00.63
– resorption, pathological K03.3
– – external K03.30
– – internal K03.31
– rotation K03.32
– shell K00.58
– spacing K07.33
– staining, intrinsic, NOS K00.8
– structure, hereditary disturbances K00.5
– supernumerary
– – canine K00.10
– – incisor K00.10
– – molar K00.12
– – premolar K00.11

– supplementary K00.1
– transplant, failure and rejection T86.8
– transposition K07.34
– Turner's K00.46

Toothache NOS K08.80

Torticollis
– congenital (sternomastoid) Q68.0X
– psychogenic F45.81
– spasmodic G24.3

Torus
– mandibularis K10.00
– palatinus K10.01

Toxoplasmosis B58.8X

Transplant failure and rejection T86.–
– bone T86.8
– bone-marrow T86.0
– skin (allograft) (autograft) T86.8
– tooth T86.8

Transposition, tooth K07.34

Treacher Collins syndrome Q87.04

Trichinellosis B75.XX

Trichuriasis B79.XX

Trigonocephaly Q75.03

Trisomy
– 13 Q91.7X
– 18 Q91.3X
– 21 Q90.VX

Tuberculosis, tuberculous
– due to HIV disease B20.0X
– jaw A18.00
– lymphadenopathy, facial and cervical A18.2X

Tuberculosis, tuberculous (*continued*)
– mouth A18.8X
– temporomandibular joint A18.00 M01.1

Tuberculum, tubercula
– abnormal K00.27
– occlusal K00.24

Tuberosity, enlargement K06.1

Tularaemia A21.–
– ulceroglandular A21.0X

Tumour
– acinar cell M8550/1
– acinic cell M8550/1
– basal cell NOS M8090/1
– benign NOS M8000/0
– carotid body M8692/1
– cells
– – benign M8001/0
– – malignant M8001/3
– – uncertain whether benign or malignant M8001/1
– embolus M8000/6
– epithelial NOS
– – benign M8010/0
– – malignant M8010/3
– giant cell, of bone
– – malignant M9250/1
– – NOS M9250/3
– glomus M8711/0
– granular cell
– – malignant M9580/3
– – NOS M9580/0
– Grawitz' M8312/3
– histiocytic D47.0X
– malignant NOS M8000/3
– mast cell D47.0X
– melanotic neuroectodermal M9363/0
– metastatic M8000/6
– mixed
– – malignant M8940/3
– – NOS M8940/0
– – salivary gland type NOS M8940/0
– mucoepidermoid M8430/1

– NOS M8000/1
– odontogenic
– – adenomatoid M9300/0
– – benign M9270/0
– – calcifying epithelial M9340/0
– – ghost cell M9302/0
– – malignant M9270/3
– – NOS M9270/1
– – squamous M9312/0
– Pindborg M9340/0
– plasma cell, malignant, NOS C90.2X
– soft tissue, benign M8800/0
– Warthin's M8561/0

Turner's
– syndrome Q96.VX
– tooth K00.46

Twitching NOS R25.3

Typhus fever A75.VX

Ulcer, ulcerating, ulcerative (of)
– aphthous, recurrent K12.00
– gingivitis
– – necrotizing A69.10
– – – acute A69.10
– – chronic K05.12
– tongue
– – NOS K14.09
– – traumatic K14.01
– traumatic, due to denture K12.04
– yaws A66.4X

Uraemia N18.VX

Urbach–Wiethe disease E78.8X

Urticaria
– giant T78.3
– pigmentosa Q82.2X

Uveoparotid fever D86.8X

Uvula
– absence, congenital Q38.50
– cleft Q35.7
– neoplasm
– – benign D10.36
– – malignant C05.2

Vaccinia B08.01

Vallecula, malignant neoplasm C10.0

Van der Woude's syndrome Q38.01

Vapours
– hot, self-harm X77.–
– NEC, toxic effect T59

Varicella B01.8X

Varices, sublingual I86.0

Vascular system, peripheral, congenital malformations Q27.–

Vasculopathy, necrotizing, NEC M31.–

Veins
– disorder NEC I87.8X
– varicose I86.–

Verruca vulgaris, oral B07.X0

Vincent's
– angina A69.11
– gingivitis A69.10

Vitamin deficiency E56.–
– A E50.8X
– B group NEC E53.–
– D E55.–
– K E56.1X

Vitiligo K80.XX

Vomiting in pregnancy, excessive O21.VX

Von Gierke's disease E74.0X

Von Recklinghausen's disease Q85.0X

Von Willebrand's disease D68.0X

Waldenström's macroglobulinaemia M9761/3, C88.0X

Warthin's tumour M8561/0

Warts, viral B07.–

Water pressure, effects of T70.–

Webbing of neck Q18.3

Wedge defect K03.10

Wegener's granulomatosis M31.3X

Whitlow, herpesviral B00.8X

Whooping cough A37.VX

Wiskott–Aldrich syndrome D82.0X

Wood preservatives, toxic effect T60

Wound
– open (of)
– – cheek S01.40
– – ear S01.3
– – eyelid S01.1
– – head S01.–
– – – multiple S01.7
– – – sequelae T90.–
– – lip S01.51
– – mouth S01.50
– – neck S11.VX
– – nose S01.2
– – periocular area S01.1
– – scalp S01.0
– – temporomandibular area S01.41
– – tongue S01.50
– operation, disruption, NEC T81.3

Xanthogranuloma D76.3X

Xanthoma, verrucous K13.42

Xeroderma pigmentosum Q82.1X

Xerostomia K11.71

Yaws A66.–
– bone lesion A66.6X
– gumma A66.4X
– joint lesion A66.6X
– ulcer A66.4X

Zinc deficiency, dietary E60.XX

Zygomycosis B46.–